VILLAGE VETS

VILLAGE VETS

Anthony Bennett & James Carroll
with Mark Whittaker

ABC
Books

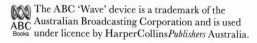 The ABC 'Wave' device is a trademark of the Australian Broadcasting Corporation and is used under licence by HarperCollins*Publishers* Australia.

First published in Australia in 2015
by HarperCollins*Publishers* Australia Pty Limited
ABN 36 009 913 517
harpercollins.com.au

HarperCollins*Publishers*
Level 13, 201 Elizabeth Street, Sydney NSW 2000, Australia
Unit D1, 63 Apollo Drive, Rosedale, Auckland 0632, New Zealand
A 53, Sector 57, Noida, UP, India
1 London Bridge Street, London, SE1 9GF, United Kingdom
2 Bloor Street East, 20th floor, Toronto, Ontario M4W 1A8, Canada
195 Broadway, New York NY 10007, USA

National Library of Australia Cataloguing-in-Publication entry:

Bennett, Anthony, author.
Village vets : one country town, two best mates and a farm
load of animals / Anthony Bennett and
James Carroll with Mark Whittaker.
ISBN: 978 0 7333 3418 4 (paperback)
ISBN: 978 1 4607 0490 5 (ebook)
Bennett, Anthony.
Carroll, James.
Veterinarians – Australia – Biography.
Veterinary medicine – Australia.
Country life – Australia.
Other Creators/Contributors:
Carroll, James, author.
Whittaker, Mark, author.
636.089092

Cover design by HarperCollins Design Studio
Front cover image by Nicholas Wilson
Back cover image by Stuart Scott
Typeset in Baskerville MT by Kirby Jones
Printed and bound in Australia by Griffin Press
The papers used by HarperCollins in the manufacture of this book
are a natural, recyclable product made from wood grown in sustainable
plantation forests. The fibre source and manufacturing processes meet
recognised international environmental standards, and carry certification.

For Sidney, Ronnie and our children,
and all the animals that have been entrusted to our care

UP TO OUR ARMPITS

James

It is dusk and a storm threatens as we flap our arms about like we're birds, whooping and urging the big black cow to go where we need her to go. We need to get her up the race and into the crush so we can save her life. She, however, is wise to our bluff. With head erect and nostrils pulsing, she wants to be far, far away. And, if she can't get there, it looks like her next favoured option will be to tango on our heads. Lightning flashes, ever closer, across the deep green flats of the Shoalhaven River. If there is thunder, we can't hear it for the wind.

Barely half an hour earlier, my new veterinary partner, Anthony Bennett, and I had been warmly ensconced in our clinic performing a delicate procedure on a cat called Ginger Meadows. Ginger was the beloved moggy of an elderly gentleman, Peter Meadows, and it was with great sadness that I'd had to tell him that Ginger had a tumour. He'd given us the go-ahead to do a biopsy to discover what sort of lump it was.

A steady hand and a high degree of coordination were required to guide a needle into the lump using an ultrasound as our navigational tool. I held the needle in place while Anthony pulled the plunger back to suck out a sample of Ginger's cells.

And then the phone rang. Trish Rosa, our dynamic veterinary nurse-cum-receptionist-cum-practice manager answered. I heard her close the call with, 'Someone will be out soon.' Not what you want to hear late on a cold August day with the wind starting to howl. 'There's a problem calving at Townsend's,' she said as she put the phone down.

As I ran through my mental checklist of everything I might need, Anthony piped up. 'I'll come with you, mate. We can take my car.' I was relieved. I'm sure it's the last thing he felt like doing, but at least he knew where the farm was.

Even though Anthony is my best mate from university, this is the first large-animal vet job we've done together in the twelve years we've known each other. For five years at uni we'd done everything in cahoots, but after that we'd gone our separate ways. I'd worked out bush in northern New South Wales, then in Wales, London and more recently in a wonderfully climate-controlled veterinary hospital in Sydney, performing delicate operations on kittens and guinea pigs, with every advanced piece of equipment imaginable on hand, and at never more than a few steps away from the tea room.

But I'd moved to Berry, a little town two hours' drive south of Sydney, to go into partnership with Anthony and now he's showing me the ropes. I haven't delivered a calf in more than four years. There isn't much demand for this sort of work in south-east London or Sydney's upper North Shore.

The blackness is fast approaching as the farm caretaker, a gentle old soul and former dairy hand called Tom, eventually manages to shoo the grunting cow into the crush while keeping a wary distance from her. Anthony squeezes the crush onto her neck to hold her fast so I can examine her. There isn't a moment to lose before this storm hits, so I go straight in – lifting the cow's tail with my right hand and sticking my bare left hand through her vulva and into the birth canal.

You might be surprised how calmly most cows accept such an indignity, but Our Girl isn't most cows. She tenses and snorts and kicks as I gently feel my way in through the narrow opening. It takes a few moments to get my bearings while I guide my hand around the slimy protrusions of bone and limb inside the huge fleshy cavity of the cow's uterus. There is a calf in there as expected.

But prod and pry as I might, I can't find the head. Or the feet.

In a calving, the front feet should come out first, followed by the head, in what we call the Superman position. When you put your hand in, you want to feel the front hooves and the nose right there near the entrance, ready to do their 'up, up and away' thing. But all I can feel here is tail.

'It's trying to come out bum first,' I say.

Often backwards calves are not a big problem. If both back legs are leading the way out of the birth canal, you can just attach a rope to the legs and pull the calf out. It's routine, with just a slightly higher risk of tearing on the way out. But bum first with the back legs pointing away from the birth canal is called a breech position. It adds a couple of degrees of difficulty.

As the winter storm wraps itself around Coolangatta Mountain, full of malicious chill that makes you think it is snowing somewhere, I've got to say I question my judgement in returning to the business of treating large animals. Why don't farmers have roofs over their crushes? And where is the tea room?

Anthony and I race to the car to grab a bit more gear as the first drops of rain begin to splash. Back at the crush I draw up the local anaesthetic for the epidural through an 18-gauge needle. This needle is so huge just looking at it makes grown men faint. But not cranky black cows, unfortunately; she thrashes about something fierce. I lift her tail and run my hand up its base, feeling for the articulations of the vertebrae where the tail meets the body. I've got to get this big fat needle directly into the space around the spinal cord of the bucking cow.

Here goes nothing.

I plunge it in and hear a tiny hiss as the bleb of local anaesthetic that was left in the hub of the needle disappears into the cow. This is good. The space around the spinal cord is under negative pressure. It's a vacuum, so it actually draws a little bit of the drug in from the needle without me pushing. Then, when I empty the contents of the syringe, I feel the tail go floppy, so I know I've hit the mark. It will deaden the back of the birth canal and vagina, but she'll still be able to feel a lot of what's going on. A more complete epidural would numb the whole area, but could cause her to lie down, and I need her to be standing.

I give her another shot to stop her pushing. I'm going to have to do a lot of pushing and pulling myself to manipulate this calf around, and if she's trying to shove the calf out, I'll lose that battle of strength. Meanwhile, Anthony has sent Tom off to get us a bucket of water. Tom comes slowly back with it slowly across the muddy yard, and Anthony pours iodine into it. I dip my arms into the dark yellow liquid right up past the elbows to sterilise them. There are no gloves for this job. My fingers will need all their feeling and dexterity for the elusive bits of calf I'll be trying to grab. I pour a few blobs of green lubricant onto my hands so they are now an ugly yellowy, greenish brown.

While the calf's bum is at the birth canal, its back legs are pointing in the wrong direction – towards the cow's head. My aim is to get hold of the back feet and pull them around 180 degrees so that they point out the birth canal instead. Before I can do that, however, I have to push the calf deeper into the uterus.

By the time I am ready to put my yellowy, greenish brown arms back in to get this calf out, the rain is coming in sideways, driving into my back. Twilight has descended early. The cow bucks and bristles. She is trying to turn her head like she wants to get a good look at the person she needs to get her revenge on. 'See you, Jimmy.'

10

I can feel that her calf is a big one and it hasn't left much room inside. I push hard on the calf, moving it back deeper into the uterus. I simultaneously pull at its feet, grunting and groaning with my neck pressed hard into the black butt of the cow. It takes all my strength, emotional and physical. These are not natural movements for me or the beast.

It almost comes as a surprise when that first leg swings back around and I am able to pull it up and out. I quickly tie a strap to it, which I leave dangling out the back so that when I get the other leg around we can start to pull.

I feel more than a bit pleased with myself. After four years away I still have it. I look over to the caretaker. Old Tom is standing off to the side and it is a bit hard to pick up the appreciative nods I am sure he wants to give me because he is battling to keep a big umbrella pointed into the horizontal rain.

I glance over to Anthony to acknowledge his professional approval. While I'm sure he knows that I know what I am doing, I still feel a need to prove it. Anthony is standing right next to me, holding the cow's tail to keep it out of my way. He is also performing another vital service: sheltering me from the south-westerly blast. My back is cold and wet but the rest of me is pretty snug. I've had my hand inside the nice warm cow with my cheek nuzzled into her angry steaming butt. Combined with the physical exertion I've been putting in, I'm relatively cosy. He's been standing still – except for some teeth chattering – taking the icy bullets for me.

So if he is giving the warm smile of professional admiration that I'm sure he wants to, I can't see it for the shaking.

'Do you want me to have a go?' he asks through those chattering teeth.

'Nah, I'll be done in a minute,' I say.

The first leg is always the hardest. I expect that now I've created more space by bringing the leg back, the second one will be easy. But

I've underestimated the physical demands of the job. Pushing and pulling against a big, difficult cow and gripping hard with my left arm at full stretch is using muscles that have rested undisturbed in city vet hospital tea rooms for four years.

I soldier on but I can feel the strength leaving my limbs.

Anthony is standing there, sheet-white, his full body shaking now.

'Do you want me to have a go?' he asks again. At least I think that's what he says. It's hard to tell amid all those vibrating teeth.

'No, I've almost got it, thanks, mate.' I'm determined to get this thing out myself, but now I start to puff and snort like the cow.

'Do you want me to have a go?' I sense that his urgency is more to do with his hypothermia than his desire to help, so I push and pull and grunt and groan some more. But he is pretty keen on getting his hands inside this nice warm cow and eventually I have to surrender.

'Yeah, you'd better take over,' I say. 'I'm knocked up. I've got nothing left.'

We swap places and I step into the full brunt of the weather. Part of me wants him to whip the calf out quickly so we can get out of here. Another part doesn't want him to do it *too* quickly. Maybe the calf knows what the weather is like out here and just doesn't want to come, because Anthony struggles a bit too. Or maybe he just wants to warm his fingers up for a few minutes before he grabs that back leg.

Either way, it doesn't take long before all of me – every last shivering, numb little bit – wants that calf out. Eventually Anthony gets the leg around and we pull out a slimy black bovine. At first it is still. We fear that it has not survived the ordeal. Anthony slaps it around the ribs and clears its airway to stimulate breathing. 'Come on, mate, wake up.' Sure enough, the forlorn slick shape on the ground splutters to life, its slippery black chest rises and falls with its rattling breath.

The clouds should have parted at this moment with a warm shaft of light cutting through to illuminate the miracle of this shiny black baby. It is the stuff of my boyhood dreams. There are few things more satisfying than bringing new life into the world, especially when the alternative is a dead calf, a dead cow and a grumbling farmer. So no matter how uncomfortable we might be, there is time to appreciate this wonder of life.

But not much time. We drag the calf quite a distance from the crush. Sometimes we'll put a new calf at the front of the crush so the mother can sniff and lick it while we clean her up, but the mum here is still too manic, snorting and dropping her head like she wants a piece of us. She doesn't know we've just saved her life. She doesn't see us as her beloved midwives who will forever share the bond of this moment.

We need to give the mother some antibiotics, some anti-inflammatories and a shot of oxytocin to help start the uterus contracting and stimulate her milk to let down. My fingers are too numb to handle a syringe, but Anthony's had his inside the cow so he manages to do it after a few fumbles. We get her ready then open up the side of the crush, making sure that we're well away. She comes out like it's the Mount Isa rodeo ... and we're the clowns. She's crazy, snorting, with wide eyes and a head that's erect and swivelling and mean. She has a go at us, even though we're safely on the other side of the rails. She patrols the perimeter, looking for a way through to get us, but then something wonderful happens.

She spots the little black lump off to the side and goes over and gives it a wary sniff. And as she realises that this is a calf, her calf, it's like the aggro just washes away with the rain. She prods and licks at it, cleaning it and probably trying to erase all evidence that Anthony and I were ever there. She's urging it to get up with her sniffs and snorts and gentle nudges of her nostrils.

Maybe I even forget the cold for a moment or two of wonder. But it's back now. The calf will soon be able to stand; however, we won't be sticking around to see it. We clean ourselves up, by which I mean we towel off our arms, but there's nowhere to change so we just throw dry towels on the ute's seats, strip off and jump in, sitting there in our undies and deciding who gets to wear the one dry pair of overalls. The only fair way is to play scissors-paper-rock. I go paper; Anthony goes scissors and gets the overalls. Darn. So I just have to sit there, willing the engine to warm up so we can get some heat running through the cabin. The cold has gone so far into my marrow that it's hard to imagine ever being warm again. As we drive out the gate, cold air still coming from the air-con vents, I realise that this is the life I've opted back into; a life of often physical labour in often miserable conditions with uncontrolled facilities and uncontrolled outcomes. Not all jobs end as happily as this one.

But it's what I want to do. I'm out here in the real world of life and death, experiencing Mother Nature in all her crazy moods. And now I'm doing it with my best mate. And it's fun. Sitting there in my undies – maybe the heat is starting to come through now as we trundle around the north side of Coolangatta Mountain and back through the roller-coasting green fields of Far Meadow towards Berry – I start to laugh.

'What's so funny?' says Anthony.

'Look at us. Imagine if someone had shown you a picture of us now when we'd first met. You'd have a run a mile.'

'I'd have run ten miles,' he says. 'I was very fit then.'

We laugh, a little hysterically perhaps, all the way home.

THE RUNNING OF THE BULLS

Anthony

Before the first day of university, all the new students were loaded onto a bus and taken to the university farm on Sydney's south-west fringe. Everybody was on their best behaviour. The guys in particular. We had just learnt that there were only twenty-five of us in the course alongside about a hundred females. So we all tried to present ourselves as eminently desirable young men, which is to say we were all acting.

By coincidence I sat near this skinny young bloke from North Sydney Boys High called James and we ended up chatting over the back of a seat for most of the drive. At lunchtime everyone went down to the cafeteria, all very earnest with our new clipboards and our air of academic solemnity. And here was this guy – a fourth-year student – with a plastic rubbish bin full of Lift mixed with white wine. He was scooping it out with a cup and trying to force it upon us.

'What is this?' we asked. He didn't have many takers; our peers were a very focused lot. James and I, however, felt sorry for him and took a drink. He was still looking lonely, so we had another. We gathered a few compassionate supporters, yet it seemed that no matter how hard we tried we could not rid him of his inner orphan.

In the afternoon, there was one of those group team-building exercises that everybody hates. We had to write a sign with our interests on it and then gravitate to other signs that appealed to us. I think I ended up under one about 'SAVING THE PLANET' and James ended up under 'BEER'. He had a girlfriend at the time so he didn't need to act eminently desirable.

The bus was a lot rowdier on the way home. And the important lesson that I took away from the day was that we weren't in high school any more. The lecturers hadn't even looked twice at our lonely purveyor of jungle juice (now a well-respected vet in the NSW Southern Highlands) who was trying to corrupt us. Nor were we in the world of paid work and bills and responsibility. We were at university, and while we knew there was a lot of work ahead, I also sensed that there might be a lot of fun to be had if we wanted it. I sensed correctly.

At the end of the first week there was a function called a keg. This one had the theme: Beer, Pies and Bull – 'All the beer you can drink, all the pies you can eat and all the mechanical bull you can ride.' At $10 a head, no poor student could refuse.

It was held out the back of the main vet faculty, an old brick-and-sandstone building with gargoyles, Latin inscriptions, battlements and the stale smell of years of learning. Walking through the building to get to the courtyard out the back, you couldn't miss the rich history. On the right was the original veterinary lecture theatre, the oldest such place in Australia. Then you walked down a hallway lined by dark wooden display cabinets filled with specimen jars and old instruments resembling medieval torture tools – horrible-looking things that would give you the shivers if you weren't racing to get to the beer, pies and bull.

The faculty had its own icebox for running a keg. It was as temperamental as a bear with a sore thumb and just two years later I would be initiated into the dark arts of operating that big white box with beer lines running through it. But at this innocent time of life, all such things were mystery and wonder.

It had just gone dark, maybe about 9 p.m. The bull was bucking and thrusting in the ring and the boys had gathered on one side of the courtyard, not yet having imbibed enough to bring them back towards the girls. We were standing over by some permanent cement-slab tables when a bunch of older guys approached us. They were third years. So even though they were as nondescript as us in their T-shirts, shorts and hiking sandals, they were still accorded the great respect that went with their vast experience.

There were about four of them and they encircled our little group of six. James was there, as well as four of our new acquaintances: Izzo, Graham, Joe and Mitch.

'We've got a very important thing to talk about,' the leader said in a serious but quiet voice, checking over his shoulder. 'We've been watching you,' he said, addressing all six of us with gravity. 'You've been nominated to be a part of NROC.' He pronounced it 'en-rock', and paused to let the magnitude of his offer sink in. 'One of the oldest and most prestigious clubs at the University of Sydney. You need to follow us immediately. Bring your drinks if you want, but we all need to go now. Don't tell anyone where you are going. Just follow us.'

How could we not accept this distinguished offer? My head was spinning with excitement. *Wow! It's like Dead Poets Society.* We formed into single file behind him and another guy, while two others fell in behind us. We were bookended as we wove our way out of the party, through the faculty, past the torture devices and preserved animal parts, and out to the front of the building. After walking through the ornate Grecian portico, we turned left into a garden that extended around the side. The path was narrow and dark. *Holy moly, what are we doing here?*

'Where are we going?' someone asked.

'What exactly is Enrock?' somebody else inquired, the concern evident in their voice.

They got no answer.

As we went around the side of the building, the noise of the party returned. We were only about 30 metres away from everyone else, but we were hidden and it was dark. The leader halted the nervous procession. 'Rightio. NROC. It's the oldest club in the university and you should realise what an honour it is to be chosen. Now get your clothes off.'

'What?'

The third years were suddenly all stripping. I had the sinking feeling that I'd just made the worst decision of my life.

'What is this? You've got to be kidding,' someone mumbled. I couldn't see James's face or that of any of the others in our group. I could just sense the fear. We were barely past remembering each other's names and asking, 'What school did you go to, again?'

The leader was down to his underpants by this time. 'NROC. It's the Nudie Run Organising Committee. Start running!'

We were bookended. If we were to get out of this, we'd have to push past a bunch of nude guys. That would be too weird. What was almost as weird was that we all simultaneously came to a spontaneous, unspoken agreement. We started tearing our clothes off. None of us had done anything like this before. Yet we were instantly united by our common lack of dignity.

I was wearing hiking boots with laces that had to be unhooked, so I was slower than the others. I didn't want to be the goose running through the crowd a minute after all the others had gone through.

'Can you wait,' I pleaded. 'C'mon guys. Back me up here.'

They waited and after we'd all stripped down we dumped our clothes in a pile on the edge of the path. Naked, we moved down the dark dirt track to the lights, the music, the people. It was like being in a quiet, dark bubble observing the chaotic world outside. And then our wise elders took off … and we followed. The single line fanned out. I remember running. Faces looking at us, too shocked to register any expression. Just stunned. They weren't laughing and they weren't screaming.

Just as we had never been on a nudie run before, our fellow first years had never seen one either. We sprinted. The adrenalin pumped. *What am I doing here?* I saw lecturers. *Is this the end of my career before it even begins?* I saw a knowing smile on one of their faces. *They've seen this before.*

I ran hard – weaving, stepping, brushing past innocent bystanders. Straight at the cement tables. *I'm going over this.* In one leap I was there, my hands in the air in absolute exhilaration, and then I was back into the historic corridor, under the Grecian portico and out into the darkness of the garden. The quiet. But it was different now. Everyone was so charged up, so exhilarated. It was the most amazing thing. I tried to get my clothes back on but struggled with all the hilarity and high-fiving, and the realisation that: *Gosh, these are probably going to be my mates. I'm in a different world now.*

Uni is a mind-altering experience.

Despite the euphoria I returned, sheepish, to the keg. *How is this going to be received?* But as we entered I detected only laughter and hooting. Everybody was on board. No one was offended. That was a relief. I felt stone-cold sober.

On Monday at lectures we couldn't look each other in the face without giggling. *Man, that dude is hairy.* It was a great icebreaker.

And that Monday was the day we got our hands on our first animals. Our course had been newly restructured, cutting out a lot of the biology and physics of first year so that we went straight into anatomy. We walked into the classroom and there were twenty dead greyhounds preserved in formalin lying on individual work stations. The sight was confronting and the smell added a few degrees of challenge. It was a combination of what I now know to be formaldehyde with a hint of what I already knew was rotting flesh. The blood gets drained from the dogs and the preservative formaldehyde is pumped in, but they can't get it to all parts of the body so a little bit of flesh tends to rot. The dogs had been frozen but were now defrosted and damp.

Greyhounds are such muscular, well-defined dogs that they are great for learning anatomy. But we were a bunch of kids. And we wouldn't have been doing vet science if we didn't love animals. Suddenly we were being asked to process all this death.

Everyone had brought along their little dissection kit that we'd bought with our textbooks before the semester. The lecturer instructed us on how to attach the scalpel blade to the handle and where we were to make our first cut. I looked at the fawn-grey dog in front of me, damp and smelly with the colour drained away.

It was easy to freak out. I could hear the hubbub of my classmates' moans and scared giggles. It was a threshold moment. One guy put his scalpel down and walked out of the room and out of the course. We never saw him again.

We were teamed in pairs and I was with a big guy called Pat who wore glasses and had a comb-over bowl haircut.

'Do you want to make the first cut?' Pat asked me.

'No ... do you?'

'Yeah, I don't mind,' he said. 'I'll do it. I'm not scared.'

'Okay, you go for it,' I said, admiring his nerve.

But as he moved in to slice the animal over the shoulder (we were studying the front leg) I noticed that his hand was flapping like a fresh-caught fish.

A POTENTIALLY LOVESICK PUPPY

James

In fourth year, all the vet students lived on campus out at Camden for half the year. It was like being on school camp for six months. It wasn't cheap, but you got all the chips you could eat. It was the best time. You'd do lectures in the morning and then, say, pregnancy-test cows in the afternoon. Every night we'd be doing something together, whether that was touch footy, trivia, pouring cold water on girls in the shower, setting fire to beds, eating chips till your belly exploded or having cold water poured on you in the shower by the girls. There was always something happening. Anthony and I even invented a sandwich – the Toasted Bread Sandwich; two pieces of toast around another piece of bread with loads of butter. Beautiful.

The way it worked then, you did your final exams at the end of fourth year. Even though we still had a year until we graduated, that was to be spent doing practical work at vet clinics. So, having lived in each other's pockets for six months, this was going to be the last hurrah. We were big on fancy dress, so we decided that each of our final exams should have a dress code. The horse exam had a horse theme, so someone brought in a saddle and did their exam sitting on that. Most of us just wore moleskins and RM Williams.

The cow exam had a bogan theme. Pigs was cross-dressing. The less said about my outfit the better, but I can tell you that Anthony looked rather fetching in a short black miniskirt and a black midriff singlet with the words 'Fashion Is A Virus' printed on it. The final exam, birds, had a formal theme so it was all bow ties, tuxedos and ball gowns. We entered arm in arm, and I'm sure the elderly exam supervisors at the front of the room were pleased with the change from the day before. No one had ever taught us boys how to sit properly with miniskirts on.

During all those years at uni, I worked in a hospital pushing beds and cleaning floors, and I also worked in a call centre as one of those annoying market-research types. So between third and fourth year I had saved enough pennies to travel to North America and work as a photographer, standing at the top of chairlifts at a ski resort. But you had to leave all that behind going into fifth year because of the requirement to do ten one-month long rotations through various clinics across the state. There was no time for paid work.

The final year starts in December. It was a shock. We were used to 130 of us moving from class to class together then having luxurious three-month holidays. But no sooner had we finished those final exams than the class dispersed across the state, having to front up in respectable clothes to work.

Both Anthony and I had chosen to do our first three months at the university's own clinic at Camperdown in inner Sydney. So we got to ease ourselves into it. Unlike a lot of our fellow students, neither of us had ever worked in a vet clinic before. It was a huge shift just getting used to being on your feet twelve hours a day. Our bums had been hardened from sitting at uni, now we all complained about how much our feet hurt. Whenever we entered a room in a group, if there was only one chair we'd all go for it like a game of musical chairs. It took a good six weeks to get used to standing all day.

There were a lot of students at Camperdown and relatively few animals, so it was an easy start. We got used to the hard floors, hard lights and the smell of antiseptic permeating every inch of those old walls. We'd all wear stethoscopes and lab coats, and I felt simultaneously kind of cool and like a big poser – hiding behind this medical façade with my pockets weighed down by pens, thermometers and other paraphernalia. A head full of knowledge and very little idea how to apply it.

The clinic was like two clinics in one: an ordinary vet clinic for the people of the city's inner west where we did the usual vaccinations, spays and broken bones; and a referral hospital where complex cases were sent to specialists, so we could find ourselves helping with complex pelvic fractures or spinal surgeries.

The resident surgeon, Dr Geraldine Hunt, was a real character. Away from surgery she'd attend social functions and always enjoy a beer with her students. But in surgery what she said went and when she said jump we leapt. Geraldine was a pioneer of a type of liver operation called portosystemic shunt surgery. We got to see and help with a few of these, whereas most vets would be lucky to see one in their whole career. It was an intense spectacle of anaesthetic and surgical expertise that Geraldine made look easy, but it was always challenging for the assisting student. The student's role was to retract the liver using an instrument that looked a lot like a metal kitchen spatula. There was always tension in the air and Geraldine was usually the only one talking, 'That's it. Hold the retractor there and don't move!' This would cause you to freeze, usually at a particularly taxing angle for your forearm. Fear of making a mistake would take over. I remember concentrating so hard on staying still that I forgot to breathe. I had to force myself to inhale, exhale, relax. Forty-five minutes is a long time to hold a pose but fear is a wonderful motivator.

Another time, calm but firm, she asked, 'Could you pass me the medium-curved Metzenbaum scissors?' Before me was an extensive tray of instruments. Years of surgery pracs meant that I knew what everything was called, but in the heat of that moment all the instruments looked remarkably similar. A moment passed. I panicked and decided on a pair of scissors that might be them.

'If I wanted Mayo scissors I would have asked for them. Try again.' Most of Geraldine's face was obscured by mask, hat and surgical attire, but her eyes said she was not impressed. Somewhere in there though, I think there was also a hint of enjoyment. She was a cat and I was her mouse.

I composed myself and picked a different pair, glancing at another student who confirmed with her eyes that I was now on the right track.

'Thank you,' Geraldine said curtly. A silent sigh of relief came from everyone in the room.

One day one of our classmates, Amanda, rushed into the treatment room, which acted as a bit of a hub for the clinic, where students would congregate to find interesting things to do. 'Oh my God, I can't go back out there,' Amanda said. 'Please, someone save me.' It didn't seem like anything was too badly wrong, though. She could hardly stop laughing.

'What's up?'

'There's a guy out there with a dog that's got conjunctivitis. He kept asking me if it was contagious to humans.' She paused here to ease her hyperventilation. 'And I told him it shouldn't be, and he asked me if I was sure that it wasn't chlamydia. I told him that dogs didn't get chlamydia. Cats did but it wasn't the same as the human version of the sexually transmitted disease. And he goes, "Are you sure it's not chlamydia?" "Positive." "You see, like, 'cause I've got chlamydia myself and sometimes …"'

Amanda stopped here and had to steady her breathing and wipe the tears from her eyes, 'And he goes, "Sometimes the dog licks me down there you know, like, on my private parts, like, when I'm asleep."'

By this time Amanda had curled herself over on the floor and was having difficulty getting the story out. We listened, gobsmacked. But she really was refusing to go back out to see the client. 'I'll give $10 to anyone who goes out there to see him for me.'

She got no takers. We were all laughing too hard.

'Twenty bucks,' she said. 'I can't go back out.'

There were probably ten of us there and we all felt the need to take a walk along the corridor and peer through the crack in the partially open door to see this guy. He was about twenty-five, unshaven and rough looking. But he was showing a lot of affection towards the Staffordshire at his feet.

'Please, I can't go back there.' Amanda begged.

In the end, Heidi, a fierce South African clinician who was Amanda's supervisor went out to complete the consult. When the man started to ask about chlamydia again, she said, 'Stop! I've heard your story. It's not chlamydia, but you do really need to stop the dog from doing that, and you should see a doctor about getting that sorted!'

101 DEAF DALMATIANS

Anthony

The Dalmatian pups were cute as, with floppy ears, black spots, blue eyes and electrodes attached to their skulls. Their owner had brought them to the university clinic, wanting us to test their hearing. So we'd taken the cuddly bundles of spots to a quiet, bare room with dull lino flooring. We'd knocked them all out with a brief anaesthetic then hooked them up for what is called a BAER (Brainstem Auditory Evoked Response) test. You put the electrodes on their heads and earphones on their ears. A series of beeps is pulsed through the earphones, then, if the dog can hear, electrodes pick up the electrical response in the brain and show it on a graph like a heart-rate monitor. If the dog is deaf, there is no response and the graph flatlines.

I was assisting the vet, Kate, with the procedure. She didn't say much as we worked our way through the seven six-week-old pups. I was unfamiliar with the machine so the readings coming through meant nothing to me.

Eventually the owner, a gruff, balding, middle-aged guy wearing a yellow pastel short-sleeved shirt, came back into the room and the puppies sparked up with their big doe eyes, looking for attention from their master.

Kate didn't bother with formalities. 'They're all deaf,' she said. 'All of them.'

'Okay then.' He turned on his heels and just walked out. I didn't understand.

I turned to Kate. 'What's that all about? Why isn't he taking the puppies?'

'They're all to be put down.'

'But you can't put them down just because they're deaf.'

She gave me a look that said, 'Yep, that's what we have to do.'

'We'll find them a new home.'

'No you can't,' Kate said. 'If the client has specified that he wants them euthanased, then we have to euthanase them.'

'Why does he want them put down?'

'He's a breeder and he's trying to protect his genetics.'

Dalmatians have a susceptibility to deafness, especially the ones with blue eyes, the same as white cats and other animals with less pigment.

'Can we say we put them down but really re-home them?'

'No, that's illegal. We have to do it.'

'Can we call him and ask if we can re-home them?'

'No. He's a breeder and he thinks that if word gets out that he's had a litter of deaf puppies then everyone will know his dogs are carrying that defective allele.'

I helped put those beautiful little pups down. It was horrendous. Not the euthanasia itself. Most of us were reconciled during the course to the inevitability that euthanasing was a necessary part of our job. But this was euthanasing them just to protect a human's financial interests. That rocked me.

This happened towards the end of our three months at the university clinic. James and I then stuck together during a month of artificial insemination and embryo transfers at Camden and then another month doing horses, but after that we went our separate ways.

As far as we knew, we'd never work together again.

ZOMBIE SHEEP AND FLYING CATS

James

I was a bit of a sickly kid. I had bad asthma when I was little and was always down with some respiratory disease or other. So I saw a lot of doctors and was fascinated by medical stuff. Right from the beginning I knew what I wanted to be when I grew up and it sure as anything wasn't a doctor. I hated those guys for what they put me through. But I loved the idea of medicine and I also loved animals.

Pretty much every photo of me as a kid has me with a dog or a cat or both. So I can't ever remember wanting to be anything but a vet.

We lived in a beautiful Queenslander right on Moreton Bay. Mum – Peg Carroll – was a nurse and Dad – David Carroll – was a mechanic. He used to work at home, and with Mum at work a lot, I was largely raised by Dad in the workshop, handing him tools, learning the intricacies of the internal combustion engine and tradesman-like language. Dad rarely swears, except when he's working, and some of that rubbed off on me, much to Mum's disgust.

My first pet was Bob the Dog, an old cattle dog who'd come off my uncle's farm because he was no good at rounding up cows. He was a great friend even if he'd get a bit cranky when I pulled his tail or his ears or stuck my finger in his eye.

It was a different time. Dogs were still roaming the streets. And even though Bob was locked in, he had a knack for getting out. Not that he did anything once he won his freedom. His idea of a good time was to go and lie in the middle of the road so all the cars had to go round him. Having grown up on a farm, when he saw the council dog catcher pull up and open his truck, he'd happily jump straight in, as if he was going to do some farm work. Poor old Mum and Dad would have to claim him back and rebuild the fence. I remember once when Dad couldn't find the dog, he went out the front only to see Bob jumping in the back of the council truck about a hundred metres away. This was Bob's second trip to the pound that month, and Dad wasn't happy. 'We can't afford to get this dog out again,' he said, exasperated. I was only about three at the time and I thought he was dead serious. Everyone else knew Dad was so soft he'd never leave Bob at the pound.

Having recently learnt about the miracle of photocopying I put forward the idea of just making our own money using a copier. Everyone laughed and Dad said not to worry, he'd sort it out. The next day Bob was back and the fence was fixed again.

Then there was our pet cat Smokey. Smokey was a quiet animal who would occasionally get a crazy glint in his eye. Often after eating fish. Smokey had a track where he'd run up the big steps at the front of the house, in the front door and then do a crazy lap of the house before leaping out the window onto the garage doors which cantilevered upwards when they were open. He'd then run along the garage roof, onto the hedge and off he'd go to maybe do another crazy lap. Except every so often the garage doors wouldn't be open. So Smokey would leap out the window and fly splendidly through the air until he hit the hard concrete driveway.

He went to the vet a few times over that, mainly with leg injuries, but I can't help thinking it didn't do his brain any favours. One day he went missing and we found him under the car. Dad took him to the vet who diagnosed him with a brain tumour and that was it for poor old Smokey.

By that time Bob the Dog had gone too. I was told Bob returned to my uncle's dairy farm where he lived out his days. (In later life I confirmed that he really did go there and it was not one of those proverbial 'trips to the farm'.)

Mum and Dad shared a dream to live on a farm. And when I was about six, they took the plunge, sold the house, got a mortgage and bought a sheep property near Wee Waa in northern New South Wales. It was probably the worst time in history to buy a sheep property because wool prices were at near record highs when they did it, but soon crashed at the same time interest rates ballooned and drought moved in.

As a kid, such matters were irrelevant. All I knew was that I was in some sort of paradise, surrounded by animals and freedom. And I got to drive a car.

Our house was 7 kilometres from the front gate where the school bus stopped. In the morning, my older brother or sister would drive the restored Ford Prefect due east into the rising sun, having to dodge the kangaroos that feasted on the sorghum Dad had planted along the driveway. The roos would scatter before us three kids in the white fridge on wheels with no seatbelts.

In the afternoon, when the risk of roo collision was gone, I'd sometimes be allowed to drive it home. My sister, Jenny, taught me. I was so short I'd have to go under the steering wheel to press the clutch in and wrestle with the two-foot-long gearstick with a little ball on the end, before climbing back up onto the seat. It didn't matter that I couldn't see where I was going because it was pretty flat and there wasn't too much to hit.

One day, Dad was fencing the paddock where the ewes were lambing and was halfway through digging a strainer post hole when something went wrong and he had to come home. When he returned to the fence next morning, he found two dirty little newborn lambs about a metre down the hole. He pulled them out. One was pretty good but the other was at death's door. Dad's a soft touch, so he thought he'd nurse them along and give them to us for something to do. Miraculously, we brought the sick one back from the dead and we called him Lazarus. We called the other one Lucy.

We hand-fed them till they were old enough to rejoin the flock. On a day when Dad had all the wethers in the yard for docking and marking, we put Lucy and Lazarus in with the mob and opened the gate for them all to go streaming back out to the paddock to their freedom. Amid all the chaos of the jittery sheep and dogs yipping away, Lucy and Lazarus made it about 50 metres before they dropped out of the flock, turned to look at us, and came running straight back. We never got rid of them from the home paddock.

My chores in the afternoon included feeding the dogs. And every time I put the food in the dogs' bowls, Lucy and Lazarus heard the sound of that kibble hitting the metal and sprinted for me, thinking that they were going to be fed their lamb pellets. They were meant to just be eating grass now, but they mustn't have got the memo. I'd hear a mad bleating that rarely came from sheep, not a sound of distress or communication, but of pure, crazy excitement. They'd leap the gate and just knock down the shed door. Lazarus would head-butt me out of the way and he clearly had me covered. I was only a scrawny seven-year-old. He'd bury his head in the feed bin before knocking it over, allowing him and Lucy to gorge themselves on the scattered dog feed, oblivious to their cannibalism. I would come back at them with whatever was at hand – brooms, shovels and, later, a cattle prodder. Anything to get them out.

We had countless fights, but the better at it I got, the more cunning Lazarus became. He was my nemesis. And much to my family's amusement I'd plan over long hours how to keep him away from me and the dog food. I'd reinforce the gate and the door, but my opponent was always one step ahead. He would lie in wait for me to make the journey from the shed to where the dogs slept and ambush me. I had to learn to think like a sheep and I'm sure this experience came into play when, years later, I won the HC Belschner Prize for Wool and Sheep.

If I was learning a lot, Dad was learning more, transitioning from mechanic to farmer. He'd spent years travelling around western Queensland with our neighbour from Brisbane, Archie Campbell, who owned vast tracts of land and had farmed all his life, but all the research in the world can't prepare you for the hardships of rural life. Things got really tough after we'd been there about a year and the drought started to take hold. Feed was scarce and the sheep were starting to go backwards, but as we weren't overstocked they were holding on okay. Then one day Dad found two sheep dead. The next day there were three more.

Dad happened to be talking to the stock and station agent who asked him how things were going. Dad told him of the deaths and that he wasn't sure what had happened. There were thousands of sheep at risk and he feared the dead ones might just be the tip of an iceberg.

'Well you should talk to your neighbour, John Melton,' the agent said. 'He's one of the biggest sheep farmers in the district.' Dad was a little confused because he hadn't come across that name and he thought he'd met all the neighbours. The agent gave Dad John's address and phone number, and Dad realised that the properties did back on to one another, but to get to the Meltons' place was about a 25-kilometre drive. Dad called John and had a chat, with John saying he'd be over first thing in the morning to have a look.

When John said 'first thing in the morning', he meant it. He was governed by the sun. He rose with it and just about went to bed with it, too. He arrived with a stockman as the sun breached the horizon, and made pleasant introductions. John was a stumpy bloke, a three-pack-a-day smoker with a red nose and spider veins cracking through his face. He always looked hot and bothered.

'Right, let's go have a look at these sheep,' he said in an excited country drawl. I tagged along and watched as he surveyed the mob. 'Not too bad. Shouldn't be dying,' was his quick summation. What he didn't like was what he saw growing in the paddock.

'See this, Dave – it's a weed, and while it looks like there's still a bit of feed, there's only this bloody weed. Shit of a stuff it is. And these buggers will be eating it and they'll all be bloody dead in no time. Got to get 'em out of here quick smart.'

With that John jumped in his little Suzuki ute, about half the size of the Hiluxes that everyone else drove. 'I'll be back in a few hours. Got to make some calls,' and off he sped in the clunky little vehicle, which, like all John's machinery, was never more than a few revs away from breaking down. Maybe he saw the benefit in befriending a mechanic, but whatever his motives, we soon saw the results.

Within a few hours he was back with a team of stockmen and a plan to get the sheep out on the stock route – that vast network of thoroughfares designed for cattle and sheep to be walked all over the country, but which, in the age of cattle trucks, now offers a safety valve against drought. Dad and my eldest brother, Simon, had them out there on the 'Long Paddock' for what seemed like an awful long time. It was tough for Dad, Simon and the sheep, but better than the inevitable death that awaited the flock at home.

When you're in a hole that deep, you remember the people who pull you out and John Melton is someone our family will be forever indebted to.

During that time, I got exposed to some of the even less fun aspects of raising animals. I remember one day on the stock route Dad was trying to find some grass for the sheep. Skinny lambs ran around their skinny mothers all battling to get some nutrition out of the brown stubble sticking out of large patches of bare earth. Even as a kid I knew the animals were under stress and I knew Dad was too.

One of the ewes had cancer – a whopping pendulous growth on the end of her ear. Conventional farming wisdom would have been to cull the ewe because the mass was infected and fly-blown, but she had a young lamb at foot and Dad couldn't afford to lose any sheep. We wanted to at least get her through long enough to wean the lamb. We caught the ewe that night and Dad cut off the ear tip. The smell of the Dettol and the sound of her brief sharp bleating remains scarred into my mind. The ewe survived; however, given what I know now, the cancer would most likely have spread and she would have died a few years later.

Another one of the problems we had was fly strike – when flies lay their eggs in the flesh of living sheep. The smell of fly strike and the chemicals you use to treat it haunt me more than Dettol. It's an awful, awful smell. The drugs back then were way more effective than now, but way more dangerous for people. I remember one day we had the chemical everywhere and I complained that it was burning my hands. John Melton turned to me and said, 'You Carrolls are soft. We used to drink a bit of arsenic every day. Made you healthy.'

John was always ranting against our softness, while his wife was always telling him to shut up. 'You're all bloody soft, you Carrolls. It's just a cut. Bit of blood never hurt anyone.' He was a real character. Mellowed as he aged, though. Gave up the smokes and the arsenic.

While this was a really tough time, it also produced some of my happiest memories. But not so happy for Mum and Dad: juggling the drought, rock-bottom wool prices and a 23.5 per cent interest-rate bill. Eventually they succumbed. They would have been better off going bankrupt but were too proud for that, so they sold the place, paid all their debts and left with nothing. It was a disaster for the family.

We said goodbye to our horse, Thirsty, and to Lucy and Lazarus. We left our working dogs, Joe and Sally, but we kept the runt of their litter, Scrawny. None of us wanted to move to Sydney, but my uncle had offered us cheap rent on a house in Ashfield and when you've got no money your options are limited. And just to top it all off the Ford Prefect carked it on the drive down.

When I started school at St Francis Xavier at Ashbury I had to wear my old yellow and brown Wee Waa uniform for a while because Mum couldn't afford the new one. All the other kids were in dark and light blues. I didn't complain because I knew the dire financial predicament we were in. The early '90s were a tough time economically for a lot of people.

I was one of only four or five Anglo kids at that school. So it was a bit of a shock coming from Wee Waa where there was a strict monoculture. For a lot of the kids, English was their second language. I helped some of them learn to read and write. It was a big change.

Mum went back to nursing and Dad went to work as a mechanic for someone else. It was tough for him. He was pushing fifty and he took what had happened pretty hard. We'd owned a waterfront house in Brisbane that would be worth a mint today. They'd gambled on a dream and lost everything. But deep down, he never gave up that dream.

None of us were happy. My sister, Jenny, had had great friends in Brisbane, and she'd made great friends in Wee Waa, and now she'd been uprooted again and she didn't like it. My eldest brother, Simon, started studying law at Sydney Uni, but as money was tight he had to work long hours to pay for it so he ended up stopping his studies to work full-time. Poor old Mum was the rock. She just kept working away. My middle brother, Dennis, went to school, and I was the youngest so the least affected, but even as a ten-year-old I was well aware of the difficulties.

It was around this time that Scrawny, the reject working dog, got sick. We took her to the vet at Croydon Park who diagnosed her with kidney failure. She was only a few years old. It's a rare condition in dogs, and the vet hoped that it was an acute case that might respond to treatment. Dad was always close to the animals and took great solace from his dog. So Mum and Dad spent money they didn't have trying to save Scrawny. They paid for blood transfusions and other treatments, but Scrawny didn't respond. In hindsight it was probably congenital. Being the runt of the litter, she would not have been destined to survive in the natural scheme of things.

I remember leaving for school one morning while Scrawny was sitting at the front door with the light streaming through the Federation-era glass like it was a cathedral. She lay there looking finished. She'd had enough. I knew she had an appointment at the vet that morning, and even if the grown-ups hadn't said as much, I sensed that she wasn't coming home. As I said goodbye I looked into her sad eyes and saw blank submission. The spark was gone; replaced with a dull, grey listlessness that in future years I would see in many old dogs when their time was up. Tough as it was, I knew it was for the best.

A THREE-LEGGED ANIMAL WITH A SPARE

James

Dad rebuilt the Ford Prefect and eventually he and Mum rebuilt their lives. Dad went back into business for himself and they bought their own house in Ashfield. By this stage I'd finished primary school and got myself into a selective high school, North Sydney Boys, which I loved.

My sister and brother both got to use the Ford Prefect when they were going to uni but the gearbox had given up the ghost by the time I got my Ls and the old car cluttered the driveway of our house for a while. Dad still has it and assures me he will restore it again.

When I was fourteen, the champion working dog that belonged to our old friends the Meltons in Wee Waa had pups. They brought a black-and-white one down and gave it to us. He was a hairy kind of dog, a border collie crossed with a huntaway, which is a New Zealand breed of sheep dog very like a border collie.

He was nominally my dog and I called him Toby. Toby the Wonder Dog.

Toby was as smart as all get out. The life of the party, always the centre of attention who hung with anyone. He was a once-in-a-lifetime kind of dog.

I also had a black mini lop rabbit called Jack, which was a poor choice of pet because after a while we figured out all the wheezing and sneezing I was doing was caused by an allergy to rabbits. Dad built Jack a hutch and we'd let him out so that he could graze the backyard. Jack didn't have a lot of personality but he was adventurous and would poke his head into everything. Then we'd have to catch him to put him back in his hutch, which was difficult because Jack was both shy and fast, and I was both slow and wheezy anywhere around him. But it didn't take long for Toby the Wonder Dog's breeding to come to the fore. He figured out how to herd Jack back into his hutch. I never had to touch Jack for the next two and a half years – at which point the neighbour's dog got him in the middle of the night.

Mum and Dad never lost the dream to return to the land and kept their eyes open for a new place. They heard about a property at Bundarra in northern New South Wales whose previous owner had gone to jail for growing a huge marijuana crop and, suffering a severe psychosis, had killed himself. The property went to auction and they picked it up for a bargain price. We quickly learnt that there's no such thing as a bargain when it comes to farming. Bundarra was tough granite country with hard winters. The previous owner hadn't worried too much about the fences, the shearing shed was actually a marijuana drying shed and the house looked like it had been built by someone smoking the stuff. But at least the country could produce a really nice superfine wool and turn off some beef.

So when I finished high school and went to uni, Mum and Dad packed their bags and went back on the land, leaving me in the capable hands of Toby the Wonder Dog. He was ridiculously obedient. You could tell him to sit somewhere and he'd still be there two hours later. I did everything with Toby. He'd come to barbies and woo everyone he met. He used to love shaking hands, he had this trick where he would shake your hands with one paw and then I'd say, 'Other paw,' and he'd give you the other one. Everyone loved it. I would have taken him to lectures if they'd let me.

One day when I was in second year at uni and Toby was about six or seven, he started limping. I felt around his foot looking for a burr or a thorn. Nothing there. I ran my hand up his leg and found a lump on his left radius – the lower part of his front leg. *Shivers, this isn't good.* I took him to the vet up the road at Enfield, Jim Allen, a tall, slightly built older gentleman who wore brown RM Williams Craftsman boots – the type intended for farmers but usually worn by city people, including me. Jim put Toby on the table, took his temperature, ran his hand up the leg and prodded around the lump. He gave it to me straight. 'It's not good. It's most likely going to be bone cancer.'

Jim X-rayed the lump and Toby's chest, confirming the diagnosis. He told me that the options were limited. There was amputation followed by chemotherapy, or there was amputation alone. If we did nothing, euthanasia would soon be the only option. The average survival time with amputation alone was six months, he said. With amputation and chemotherapy it was twelve months.

Funds were tight during those uni days, and the chemo was very expensive and only offered an extra six months of life, so I decided the best I could do for Toby was to have the leg amputated. People are always touchy about having a three-legged dog. They think their pet is going to hate it. They're wrong. Dogs are resilient; you chop 'em off and they don't care. We've got a specialist surgeon, Eugene Buffa, who visits Berry to perform operations for us. He describes it thus: 'Dogs are a three-legged animal with a spare.'

Toby came back from the vet a three-legged dog. It hardly slowed him down at all, though he found it difficult to walk at human pace with three legs. He could either go fast or really slow but he couldn't match my natural stride. So he ended up on a very generous rope and he'd either be a long way in front or a long way behind. He still loved shaking hands; you'd take him for a walk and he'd try to shake with everybody you talked to. One day after the operation, out of habit I said, 'Other paw.'

Toby looked down and paused, and you could see his momentary confusion, but he handed over his stump and looked pretty pleased with himself. We all laughed so he looked even more chuffed.

In a short time he became a local celebrity around Enfield. People loved the three-legged dog on the enormous old rope.

He was still mad for chasing a ball. The trouble was when he chased it on a slope with his missing leg – the front left – on the downhill side. He would normally have taken all his weight with that leg, but when he was chasing a ball, he was so focused on the task at hand that he just gave no thought to staying upright, and would routinely tumble down the hill. It took him months to figure it out. Precious months as it turned out.

Unfortunately, osteosarcoma, primary cancer of the bone, usually metastasises to the lungs. Almost six months to the day after the amputation, I noticed Toby breathing strangely. I took him back to Jim Allen, who gave him another X-ray. The cancer had spread. Normally such cancers cause coughing, but Toby's tumours were concentrated on the outside of the lungs. So he'd leaked fluid from the cancer clusters into the cavity between the lung and the chest wall, and the accumulation of fluid made breathing difficult. He couldn't expand his lungs.

Knowing that I was a student, Jim let me help with an operation to relieve him. We sedated Toby, gave him some local anaesthetic and made a small puncture below the ribs. The vet inserted a tube and immediately a steady flow of clear blood-tinged fluid started draining into a kidney dish. About a litre came out in all.

Once we'd brought him out of the anaesthetic, Toby was like new again. He chased the ball and shook hands like the Wonder Dog of old. But I knew he was on borrowed time. At least it gave me three weeks to get my head around the thought of losing the best dog ever. Inevitably, the chest filled again.

I was away on prac work when they phoned me up and told me Toby was in respiratory distress. It was time to put him to sleep. I was devastated, but it wasn't fair to expect Toby to wait at home for me to come back. My brother Dennis took him in to Jim.

Poor old Toby the Wonder Dog.

WHEN PIGS FLY

Anthony

We were almost halfway through our final year of uni before I went to my first private practice at Gloucester, three and a half hours north of Sydney. I'd given up my part-time job as a waiter at the local sailing club so I had no money. I chose Gloucester on the basis that I had family out there and therefore free accommodation.

The vet, Arthur 'Otto' Pointing, came out to meet me on my first morning. He was shortish, with a thick neck, a thick beard and giant forearms like those of a man who'd done a lot of hard work.

He looked me up and down and without being overly friendly about it said, 'Pleased to meet you. Jump in the car. Let's go.' As we drove to our first job of the day, he explained that it was usually a three-vet practice but his two colleagues had just left. We were on our own. We drove from farm to farm, dealing with all the problems as they mounted up. I felt absolutely hopeless. I'd never been in private practice before. I didn't know how to put catheters in, how to take blood. Struggling to do the work of three vets, Arthur didn't have time to teach me. Nor did he have time to be critical of me either. But I tried as hard as I could to learn. I was just an extra set of hands, helping wherever I could.

One day we got back to the clinic at 8 p.m., absolutely beat. An elderly widow came in with a little Maltese terrier, called Trixie. The little white ball of fluff had lost her appetite and was excessively thirsty, dehydrated and lethargic. 'She's weeing all over the place,' said her bent-over owner. 'And smell her breath. It's got a real funny sweet smell to it.'

'What do you think, Anthony?' Arthur asked.

'Could be diabetes, Arthur,' I said.

'Sounds like it to me.'

Yes! I'd got something right.

For dogs with diabetes you need a strict regime of insulin and food, delivered on a tight timetable. Even in a big practice with plenty of vets and nurses it is difficult to treat, and we certainly weren't one of those. And Trixie was a vicious little thing. The reality of veterinary life is that savage animals are harder to treat, so they cannot get the same level of care that placid ones get. Arthur never swore, so when he grumbled about this dog it was the 'Bathplug'. But he had a really good heart. He knew what Trixie meant to her widowed owner so he gave the treatment his best shot. We'd get back from a long day on the road – we might have driven 180 kilometres to deliver a calf – and there'd be Trixie, sitting in her cage waiting for her food and insulin. Waiting to maul the hand that fed her. But we did what we could and got her a little bit better.

Arthur ended up delivering Trixie home too, driving 15 kilometres out to the widow's place to deliver the horrid little Bathplug. It was a great lesson for me in hard work and empathy.

I finished up at Gloucester and came back to Sydney to do a month at the Gladesville Veterinary Clinic. Everybody wanted to go to Gladesville. It had a huge reputation as a high-end clinic, and on top of that, the TV vet Dr Harry Cooper was a former owner. *Hey, imagine that. I wonder what it was like when he was here. I'm going to come out of this with so much experience.* The uni had a ballot system to see who got to go where and I must have come out fairly high up to have scored Gladesville. That place had an aura.

It was so up-market, with everything having to be done in such an exacting fashion that there was no way they were going to let a student near anything that could be stuffed up. The owners, Max and Barry, were fantastic mentors but the overriding thing I learnt there was that I definitely didn't want to go into small-animal practice in a big city. I wanted to become a vet because I loved animals, but the human element was really important to me too, as was getting out and about. At Gladesville you could go days without actually seeing a client. The only time you went outside was to walk animals from the main hospital to the shed.

After Gladesville, I went off to do my compulsory government rotation with a vet who worked for the Rural Lands Protection Board at Nyngan, in the state's west. I walked into the office and a slender guy of about fifty stood to greet me. 'Hi, I'm Aarn.'

'G'day, I'm Anthony. What's your last name so I can call you "Doctor" when we're with clients?'

'No, it's just Aarn. There's no first, no last.'

He told me he was retiring the day I finished, and that he'd stayed on an extra few weeks solely so I could come out and do my rotation. 'I've organised accommodation for you in the nurses' barracks. The nurses aren't there any more but you can stay there for $5 a night.'

'Great, but I would pay $10 if the nurses were there.'

'I live there as well,' he said, deadpan, giving the impression that a bunch of nurses was the last thing he'd want. 'It's the cheapest place I could get. I've got the whole place to myself.'

He told me he was a runner, so I told him I was too. I had visions of us jogging in the mornings and that I'd get to know this guy really well. I suggested we share meals too.

'No, I don't want to share meals and I'd prefer to run alone.'

Aarn was nothing out of the ordinary to look at but I soon saw that he marched to a different drum. He suggested I drive everywhere because he didn't like driving, and that was cool because I loved it. I was struck by the flatness of the land. I'd never seen that type of country before, where the horizon stretches away evenly forever, broken only by the shimmer of the heat haze. Our conversations were halted and awkward so after a few failed attempts at finding common ground, I'd occupy myself on the long drives by calculating how far away in the distance an oncoming car might be. By estimating their speed combined with my speed and the time it took to pass them, I'd figure what the distance had been when I first saw them. This was especially easy at night. My record was 17 kilometres.

One time Aarn said, 'Quick! Pull over. Right here.' He jumped out with a big plastic bag and started grabbing lucerne from the side of the road. 'This is the solution to third-world poverty,' he said as he got back in with the bag overflowing. He'd read that lucerne was highly nutritious, full of iron and protein, and could be grown almost anywhere. He took it home and microwaved it with garlic and that was his entire meal. The place smelled like rotten cabbage and as the odour wafted through the barracks I was suddenly glad he'd declined my offer to share food.

Though he didn't conform to the whole rural community thing of tough farm blokes, with their pigging, drinking and footy, he was great for me to work with.

'Can you preg-test cows?' he asked one day.

'Not well enough to be 100 per cent guaranteed, but yes I can.'

'Oh, that's good. I've got a lot of farmers who want that done. They understand that you're not crash hot at it, but they'd still like an idea.'

So we started doing the rounds and I'd hop out of the driver's seat and the farmer would come up to me, 'G'day, how's it going?', thinking I was the vet and the little guy in the passenger seat was the student.

'No, I've just driven here. Aarn's the vet,' I'd say.

'Right. So he's doing the preg-testing?'

'No. That's me.'

'So you're the vet?'

'No, I'm the student. But I'm doing the testing.'

As uncomfortable as it was, all vet students crave this kind of experience. Preg-testing is a numbers game. You have to do a lot to get the feel for it, and thanks to Aarn I was getting my numbers up.

He even teed up a stint for me with the local vet and also to go up in a helicopter to observe National Parks and Wildlife shooters culling pigs in the Macquarie Marshes. Pigs do a lot of damage to the delicate wetlands. All Australian mammals have soft-padded feet that barely disturb the soil, but introduced species have hard, cloven feet and their mere presence causes enormous destruction. Combine that with the pig's hard snout and desire to root around looking for food, and they are basically a wetland's worst nightmare.

As much as vets and rangers hate to destroy life, there really is no choice but to remove the introduced pests. It is either that or sacrifice the hundreds and thousands of native animals that rely on the wetlands for habitat. Shooting is thought to be the most humane way to eradicate them, and helicopters are needed to get the highly trained marksmen to their targets in the otherwise impenetrable country. Having done a bit of shooting with an air rifle as a kid, I was keen to see how the professionals did it

I turned up at the local airport not knowing exactly what to expect. When I went to get on board the helicopter, the clean-shaven pilot with Aviators and a big, round helmet asked, 'Would you like to be sitting inside or outside of the helicopter?'

'Definitely outside.'

They rigged me up in a harness so I could lean right out. The pilot would swoop down towards thickets of scrub. The chopper had a siren and flashing lights to flush the pigs out into the open, and once they'd break loose, we could fly sideways or forwards as the shooter picked them off with enormous bullets fired from his enormous rifle. The pigs died instantly and with very little stress.

It was quite surreal. Some pigs would take to the water and try to swim. The helicopter flew in sideways – Bang! – a giant bullet into the mother, then – Bang! Bang! Bang! Bang! – along the line of piglets behind her. There'd be a puff of blood and the pink pig would sink, disappearing from view. The entire day I did not see the shooter miss once, nor did I see a pig survive after being shot.

For all the excitement, it was very unsettling. I remember the pilot, who didn't waste a lot of energy with talk, saying, 'I started my career thirty years ago flying helicopters for people to shoot things, and now I'm finishing my career doing the same thing.'

'Where'd you start?' I asked over the thud of the blades.

'Vietnam,' he said. 'And we weren't shooting pigs.'

I didn't know what to say.

Despite the fact that the pigs fell instantly, the shooter wanted to ensure that the bullets were having the intended effect and the pigs were actually dying quickly and painlessly. He figured that having a vet student on board was an opportunity to find out. 'Hey listen. We're just going to drop you off here so that you can give them a post-mortem. Find out how they're dying.'

'Oh … rightio. A bullet I'm betting.'

I was handed a white-handled butcher's knife and a steel to sharpen it with. The pilot dropped down onto a newly shot cluster of animals and they kicked me out of the chopper.

Whump, whump, whump. Off it flew, kicking up a whirlwind of noise and confusion. Then there I was, standing in the sudden silence. The emptiness of the scene left plenty of room for my imagination to fill it with angry wounded boars brandishing foot-long tusks leaping out of the nearby bushes. The helicopter was so far away I couldn't even hear it, or the gun. And that was a noisy helicopter and an even noisier gun.

I hope they remember where they dropped me. What if they crash? The rescuers will find them but not me.

I had a bit of a poke and a prod into the dark hairy carcass of one animal, but my feet were in a couple of inches of water, it was stinking hot, ants were darting over the corpse and quite frankly I was more interested in keeping an eye on the four-foot-high reeds surrounding me than cutting up that animal. Every time the wind rustled the reeds I imagined that enormous boar storming through them. By the time the chopper came back I hadn't achieved much. 'Look, I'm not doing any more like that,' I said. 'You can pick them up and take them back to camp on the helicopter.'

And that's what we did. We dragged the pigs into a sling and tied that to the chopper with a 6-metre rope.

I did a post-mortem back at camp and found that the bullets mostly entered in the region of the shoulder, right where the shooter was aiming, and disintegrated inside the animal – which indicated a very rapid demise.

LOST IN SPAYS

James

I had my hands deep inside the yellow kelpie, performing my first ever spay – the desexing of a female animal – when I grabbed the right ovary to try and pull it out. Because the ovaries are deep inside the dog and you can't see what you're doing, I was operating by feel. But being so new at it, I didn't have the feeling. That's something you only get with experience. I knew enough, however, to know that something was wrong. I peered in as best I could. There was blood. There was uterus. There was no ovary. I realised that I had torn the ovary away from the uterus, ripping a hole in it.

Holy crap. What do I do now?

The situation was made so much better and so much worse by the fact that I was operating on my own dog. I didn't want to kill somebody else's dog, but equally I didn't want to kill my own. Not Bailey. She was brand-new. Mum and Dad had just given her to me. And Bailey wasn't just any old pup. She was the granddaughter of the dog who'd chaperoned me through my teens and early adulthood – Toby the Wonder Dog. I couldn't tolerate the thought of losing his granddaughter through my own ineptitude.

I was in the final year of uni. It was a tough time financially because I couldn't hold down a job. I'd tried to do as many of my rotations as possible near Mum and Dad's place so that I had somewhere free to stay. Bundarra is equidistant from the much larger towns of Inverell and Barraba and I'd managed to score a rotation at each of their vet clinics.

When I'd been there for Christmas at the beginning of fourth year, Mum and Dad had had a litter of puppies running around and let me choose one for a pet. There was a yellow female that seemed to be the most adventurous. She was always coming back from her forays into the wide world covered in grease and poo. I liked her spirit so I chose her and called her Bailey.

While Bailey was the granddaughter of Toby the Wonder Dog, it was a little more complicated than that. Even though Toby had been a useless working dog, because he'd been brought up in the city, he was genetically gifted. So when Mum and Dad had moved back to the country, they'd acquired an experienced working dog called Lea. Lea and Toby had had pups and two of those pups stayed on as working dogs. Buster was a female yellow kelpie and Dusty was a black-and-tan male. Their grand heritage had come shining through and they'd proven themselves to be very good at rounding up animals.

Dad was working the sheep with them one day soon after Buster had been on heat. At least he thought she'd come off heat. But amid the chaos of a lot of sheep on the move, she and her brother Dusty did the deed somewhere out of his sight. Before Dad knew it, Buster's breast tissue was showing a distinct swelling. She was about to give birth.

So Dad let me have this beautiful golden puppy. I was so excited to have a new incarnation of the Wonder Dog. I expected her to be just like her bold and friendly twice-over granddad, but whether or not it was a result of the genetic screw-up or just that every dog is different, Bailey turned out to be nothing like him.

Even though she'd appeared outgoing as a pup, as soon as I took her home with me she just wanted to hide under the blankets or lie in front of the fire. It was like she was scared of the world. It required a mind shift from me, and I was still struggling with that when I found myself operating on her to ensure that no more pups would come out of this lineage.

I had started my stint at the Barraba vet clinic and one of the vets there, Margot, who was herself only in her first year out of uni, agreed to supervise while I had a go.

Spaying a dog is a major surgery. And difficult. I'd heard older vets say things like, 'Once you can spay a dog, you can do any other soft-tissue surgery.' So I was pretty keen to get one under my belt.

We knocked Bailey out with a general anaesthetic, Alfaxan, placed a tube down her windpipe and hooked her up to the anaesthetic machine so the gasses would keep her asleep. I made the incision in her abdomen.

I would have been nervous regardless of whose dog it was, but doing the operation on Bailey added to the butterflies in my stomach. I'd done this operation once before on a cadaver at uni, and I'd assisted on one at the university clinic a few months earlier, but I'd never been truly responsible for one. As I pressed down through the skin with the scalpel, I was following my road map. I searched for the *linea alba*, which is Latin for 'white line'. It's a fusion of muscles that meet in the midline of the chest. I made a small stab there, putting me into the abdomen, then picked up the scissors to extend the cut down Bailey's belly.

Once inside, I had to fish around to find the uterus and the ovaries. Blood oozed from tissues that were already a little slippery from the fat in the abdomen. Things were difficult to grasp and manipulate. It was something like a soup in there.

A dog like a kelpie has a deep chest and small abdomen, so the uterus resides down towards the rib cage – deep inside. You find the uterus and trace along it with your fingers until you reach the ovary, which feels like a small, squishy grape. You're doing it blind. There's fat, intestines and other organs in there to confuse you.

So I felt my way along. It took a while to get my bearings. There was tension and frustration, but I eventually had that ovary in my fingers. It's attached to the kidney by the ovarian ligament, down towards the aorta and all the other serious blood vessels going to and from the heart, so you can't just bring out the scalpel and cut it off.

'Can you feel the ligament holding it in place?' Margot asked.

'Yeah, I think so.'

'Now you've got to snap that. But be careful of the blood vessels sitting right next to you there. Damage those and you're in big trouble.'

So I had the ovary pincered between my left thumb and index finger. I got my right index finger up underneath the ligament and pulled the whole unit upwards, backwards and towards the centre of the dog, while it also worked at snapping the ovary. I heard and felt a snap. My stomach jumped a little. I surveyed the scene to see if anything was wrong and then I breathed. It was all okay. The ovary and uterus were a lot more mobile now, so I pulled the whole uterus upwards and back towards me with gentle pressure. I could see it now. It looked like a piece of string with a grape at the end.

Once I had the uterus out, I put three clamps on the blood vessels that deliver blood to and from the ovary. I tied them off with a surgeon's knot that had been practised and mastered in surgery classes. Then, snip, it was done.

'Make sure everything is okay before you let it go,' Margot said. 'Once you let go it will spring back towards the kidney and it's hard to find again.'

But everything looked perfect. I released the clamp and held on carefully with some forceps. There was no blood, so I let it go and in it went. Nothing changed, no blood welled up; it all looked great. I patted myself on the back; however, there were two ovaries and I'd just done the easy one on the left. Now it was time to tackle the right with all the confidence and experience I'd just gained. It was like playing one good golf shot and thinking that now I had the game nailed.

The right ovary and kidney sit deeper in the dog and are more difficult to access. But I went in with self-assurance. I found the uterus, traced along it, grabbed the ovary and began to retract it to start the process of snapping the ligament again. This time, however, as I snapped I felt a different sensation and a different, almost inaudible noise. The uterus was now mobile but the ovary was still fixed in position. Something was wrong.

'Oh shit, oh shit, oh shit. I've torn the uterus. Margot can you scrub in and give me a hand?'

'It's okay, don't stress,' Margot had the patience of a saint. 'We'll just make a larger incision. We'll find what we need to find and get it done.'

So I cut a bigger hole in Bailey's belly. This gave us more room to work in and see what we were doing. There was some blood due to the uterus tearing, which meant that it was difficult to see things properly. Now with a big incision I had to very gently stretch the uterine ligament up just enough to give me access. I dared not attempt snapping it again for fear of further damage and bleeding. I gently got in far enough to see what I was doing and was able to get the three clamps on, with Margot helping retract everything out of the way. Painstakingly, we tied up the veins and arteries.

Then came the moment of truth. Swabbing out the abdomen, we let the tied-up blood vessels go. There was no more bleeding. Everything was okay. With an incredible sense of relief and with Margot's calm voice keeping things steady, I stitched poor Bailey up. She didn't seem to cope well with the recovery from her anaesthetic, so I stayed by her side diligently waiting for her to wake. As the first glimmers of consciousness started to come across her face and mouth, I reached down to comfort her. She looked up at me with those big woozy eyes … and bit me on the hand. Hard. It hurt a lot and I swore like a Brisbane motor mechanic, but I didn't feel anger towards her. It was very out of character for her, and besides, after what I'd just put her through, perhaps she had reasonable grounds.

A BLOODY FAST GREYHOUND

Anthony

When the infrared buzzer sounded on the clinic door and I saw the middle-aged man come in, I knew it wasn't going to be an ordinary consult. He wore a small hat with a feather in it, had a notebook and pen in the pocket of his blue-hibiscus Hawaiian shirt and a newspaper form guide hanging out the back pocket of his grey slacks, which were held up by an overworked brown belt.

'G'day, I'm Max Pringle. I wanna see the vet about me greyhound,' he said.

I was starting my very last rotation at a clinic in the Shoalhaven district. They had the contract to do the veterinary work at the Nowra greyhound track, so they saw a lot of racing dogs. When Max came in and approached the counter, it was clear that his dog had the problem which trainers hate most and which afflicts the great majority of racing dogs … it wasn't running as fast as the dogs beside it.

When the vet, Nigel, came out to see him, Max got straight to the point. 'I wanna bleed me dog,' he said. 'And I want you to do it.'

I'd heard about the practice of bloodletting before, but only as a historical oddity. I had no idea it still existed.

'No, I don't think that's a good idea,' Nigel said.

'Yeah, well he's not going any good. I think he's got some bad blood in him and we've got to get it out.'

'No, that's a bit of an old wives' tale. It's not backed up by science,' Nigel said, flicking back his long blond hair. 'There's no reason to do it. I can't do something like that to an animal unless there's a reason.'

'Yeah, well, my father did it and all the other guys are doing it. Their vets do it for them and I want you to do it. That's reason enough isn't it?'

'Look, no, I'm not going to do it. But why don't you bring the dog in and we'll have a look at him to see if we can find something wrong?'

But Max wouldn't have it. 'I know what's wrong with him and I know how to fix it. Be seein' ya.' And with that he went back through the buzzer and out the door.

The conversation had gone a bit over my head, but once Max left, the vet explained to me that there wasn't a lot of money in greyhound racing. Many of its practitioners were poorly educated battlers and a lot of their medical ideas – like bloodletting, which had been a frontline remedy for doctors from the time of the ancient Egyptians right through to the early 1800s – had managed to persist because many of their training techniques were handed down from generation to generation.

In horses there is a possibility that removing blood does improve performance. The theory is that newer red blood cells have a slightly higher oxygen-carrying capacity. When you remove blood from horses it is rapidly replaced by these new cells. But the greyhound trainers were missing one important point. Horses have an enormous number of new red blood cells waiting to be released from the spleen. Dogs do not. Removing blood from a dog simply makes it anaemic. About the last thing you feel like doing after giving blood is running a race. You didn't see Lance Armstrong donating blood during the Tour; quite the opposite really.

The greyhound track was a real eye-opener for me as I watched vets battling to re-educate trainers who thought they were doing the right thing in applying their ancient and not-so-ancient practices. And there was a lot of work to do on Max. Three days later, he reappeared at the counter, still smelling of the cigarette he'd stamped out on the path outside and the spaghetti bolognese he'd had for breakfast. In his hat and polyester slacks, he might have looked right at home at the track, but in the waiting room of a small-animal practice he stood out like a fur coat at a PETA conference.

'I need to speak to the vet,' he said. Nigel was summoned to the waiting room.

'Look,' said Max, 'I've been thinking about this bleeding. I think I can do it myself. If I just cut the dog there over the neck with a knife, that's its jugular isn't it? I can see it right there. That's all I've got to do isn't it?'

'Holy shit! You're going to cut the dog's throat,' Nigel said, letting his exasperation show. 'Do you really think that's going to make him run faster? You'd better bring him in.' Nigel was stuck in a bind. If he didn't bleed the dog, Max was going to cut the dog's throat. At least if Nigel did it the dog would be safe(ish).

Max brought the dog in. His name was Harry the Far-Cup. He was grey, sleek and tall for a greyhound, almost coming up to waist height. His back legs were so muscular that he struggled to walk without the muscles chafing. Trainers often countered this problem by applying Vaseline between the legs, and when this mixed with sweat it formed a foamy white residue. This was evident on Harry the Far-Cup's legs.

After another attempt to convince Max that this treatment wasn't going to achieve anything, we took Harry into the operating area, leaving Max calling out from the waiting room: 'Make sure you take a good amount. I want at least a litre.'

Harry had a lovely placid nature and he nuzzled into me as we sedated him. Being as lean as greyhounds are, we could see every vein, so it was a simple matter to put pressure on the base of Harry's neck to make the veins swell and bulge. Nigel placed a 14-gauge needle into the dog's jugular and attached the needle to a blood collection bag. He lowered the bag below the level of the dog and just let gravity do the work.

There was no way we were going to take a litre. That would just about kill the dog. Human donations are usually 470 millilitres. But Max didn't need to know that we were taking less than he wanted. Doing this in a backyard would be so dangerous it was hard to conceive of anybody getting away with it. At least we were doing it in a controlled, clean environment.

Nigel was going to keep the blood in case he had to do any dog transfusions in the next three weeks. Dog blood only remains good for about that long, but the beauty of it is that you can transfuse it into any dog receiving their first transfusion.

So we bled Harry the Far-Cup. We took 400 millilitres, and a few hours later Max came by to pick him up. 'You took enough didn't you? I wanted you to take a litre and a half.'

'Don't worry. We took enough.'

'I wanted you to do it properly,' Max said. 'I won't be happy if you haven't taken enough.'

I was flabbergasted at the gall of this know-nothing who thought he could tell the vet not only that he wanted the dog bled but how much he should take.

Max clipped the dog on the lead and walked it away, but I noted its head and tail were a little down and there was no spring in its step.

The following week we were at the track performing all the routine veterinary functions. I was impressed by those dogs. They were elite athletes beyond anything humans could hope to emulate. When the winners came through after the race, there was a system whereby the officials would draw a number out of a basket and if it matched the winner's number it would have to be swabbed for drugs.

These dogs might have run 520 metres in almost thirty seconds, so you'd hold the cup out for them to urinate in and what came out looked like blood. It was actually muscle fibre that had broken down in the massive exertion of the race then been excreted via the kidneys. And despite all that they were the most even-tempered of animals. They're fascinating to work with.

So we were at the track and I was really enjoying the hubbub of it all when I saw Max in the ticket-strewn public area. I was a little disappointed when I saw him change direction and head towards us with his fast little steps.

'G'day Max, how's your luck holding up?'

'Look, the dog's a bit sluggish,' he said, his face tightening to a grimace that made it look like he was thinking very hard. When he opened his mouth for a second time it was apparent that he hadn't been. 'Any chance I could get some anabolics to build him back up?'

'You don't reckon it's sluggish because it's anaemic from all that blood you wanted removed?' Nigel said.

'Nah, nah, that makes them go faster,' Max countered. 'What it needs is some steroids.'

'You do know I'm the official course vet here?'

Max looked at Nigel like he was thinking real hard again, sizing him up.

'Yeah, I'm not saying I'm gunna do it. It's just that that's what it *needs*. Maybe some more bleeding too.' And with that, he turned and scurried into the ring, pulling the form guide from his back pocket and disappearing into the crowd.

INVERELL CAESAREAN

James

I'd heard Bob's voice on the phone. It was throaty and distinctive, like he should be presenting the *Country Hour* on ABC Radio. But when I met him at the Inverell vet clinic he was quite different to what I'd anticipated. He was short and tanned with wavy hair and a few extra kilos hanging off his middle. He was chatty as he gave me a quick tour of the place, then pointed at a little mongrel in one of the cages. 'Come on, we'll spay this dog,' he said, grabbing the cage.

He arranged the gear on a tray and asked me what size gloves I wore. 'You do it, I'll watch,' he said.

I told him I'd spayed a few dogs in Barraba, but I might have omitted some of the details of Bailey's complications. Bob watched me perform probably my fourth or fifth spay and it all went smoothly. 'You're pretty good at that,' he said. 'Every spay and castrate that comes in this month, you do it. That'll free me up. Any troubles, I'll be around to help you, but I reckon you've got it.'

I knew then that this was going to be a good rotation. Experience is everything. We'd spent four years stuffing our heads with theory. What we needed was to get our hands in and do it. Bob seemed perfectly aware of how our interests collided on this matter. No one there needed to learn how to spay a dog. I did. Perfect.

The clinic was made up of Bob, his business partner Greg, and Ray, another vet. Greg was a tall, wiry guy with a hipster-style beard, long before hipsters existed. A former jackaroo, he was full of energy and really down to earth. Ray was a former ringleader of NROC who was now reformed into a hardworking vet, but still had a glint of larrikin in his eye.

Inverell is almost 600 metres above sea level so it suffers bitterly cold winter nights and mornings, but it's a long way north of Sydney so the days become spectacular and warm. It was on one such frigid morning that Bob came in cursing. 'Bloody hell, we've got a calving way up past Warialda. Why couldn't it have happened yesterday when we were up there?' He had a branch clinic at Warialda, 60 kilometres away, which was open three days a week, so naturally Murphy's Law demanded that the emergencies happened on the other days. We got in the car and drove.

Bob was an entertaining character, studious and perhaps a little more arty than you usually find in scientific professions. On the drive he told me how he was only working because he had to support his ex-wives. He also told me about one time when he was driving through a particular town and started to get severe chest pains. 'I knew I was having a heart attack but I wasn't going to stop there. It's full of hicks and inbreds. I kept driving, thinking "I don't want to die in ******." The fear of dying in that place kept me going and got me to hospital.' Some people thought Bob was cranky, but I thought he was an endearing curmudgeon.

The sun was shining warmly now and all was right with the world as we drove into Warialda and turned right, heading another 40 kilometres or so north towards the Queensland border.

We got to the place and I saw that the crossbred cattle looked in fine condition and there was not a wire out of place on the farm. The farmer, Trevor Schmidt, a white-haired guy in his sixties came out of the beautiful leafy house-garden to meet us. He led us to the yards, which were clean and well set up – shaded by the shed built onto the side. You get a vibe about a place when you arrive, and the vibe here was that Trevor was immaculate and precise, almost obsessively so.

The cow in question, an Angus-Hereford cross, had a mostly black body with a white face. She was loitering in the yard near the race. 'I found her this morning,' Trevor said. 'She's pretty crook. We keep them up near the house when they're close to calving but the only reason I noticed her was that she wasn't hanging out with the others. She was over on her own. There's been nothing showing, and I haven't seen her pushing, but she's obviously been trying to calve for a while, going by the smell of her.'

While we don't tend to wear gloves with calvings, the odour emanating from this cow, even from a distance, was bad enough to prompt Bob to pull one on. He put his gloved hand in the cow, made a worried face and started shaking his head.

He looked at me. 'You better put your hand in here James and tell me what you think.' He wasn't going to tell me. It was all part of the education. I had to figure it out myself. The farmer was in on it too, waiting for my turn to be over before asking any further questions. So I pulled on a glove and did my best not to grimace too wildly as I tried to stick my hand in. I had seen and smelled a couple of rotten calvings before, but this was by far the worst. When a calf dies inside the mother, it starts to decompose. If you don't get it out, the toxic overload eventually kills the mother as well. But the other thing about this one was that there was hardly enough space for me to squeeze my hand into the birth canal.

'The cervix is closed down,' I said. 'I can feel the calf on the other side, but there's no way we can get it out.'

'That's right,' Bob said. 'You can barely get a couple of fingers through, though your dainty little arms might fit, James.' He laughed at his joke. 'There's nothing we can do to get this calf out the back.'

The usual thing to do with a rotten calf if you can't pull it out whole is to cut it up inside the cow and then pull it out bit by bit, but with the closed cervix we couldn't reach in to do that, and even if we could, the head wouldn't fit out.

Bob turned to the owner. 'In essence, Trevor, nothing has reached into that pelvic canal to stimulate her to push, but the calf died some time ago and it's been rotting away in there. You haven't noticed her pushing because she hasn't been pushing. The cervix would have been open a few days ago, but it's well and truly closed down now. As far as she's concerned, calving is finished.'

So we stood there and looked her over while Bob thought about what to do. He eventually broke the silence. 'Look, this cow's pretty crook. There's not much we can do. Your options are three: you can hope that this calf rots inside and you can pull it out in bits over the coming week or two; you can shoot her; or we can do a caesarean.'

Trevor thought about this for a while. 'She's a good cow. She's produced some good calves. What do you think her chances of surviving a caesarean are?'

Bob shook his head and mumbled gruffly to himself. 'To be honest, three-fifths of stuff all.'

'And how much is it gunna cost?' Trevor asked.

'Well, it's going to cost a few hundred dollars.'

The farmer looked at the cow and looked at Bob. 'She's not gunna live is she?'

'Probably not. From a business point of view, you're probably throwing good money after bad.'

'All right, that being the case, I think we'll probably put her out of her misery.'

Bob looked at me then looked at his watch. We stood there in silence a while longer. In the country, the length of time you can go without saying anything – and without getting uncomfortable about not saying anything – is a lot longer than in the city. So there we were, three blokes not saying much, until Bob broke the silence. 'Look, there is one more option. James here has been hanging around for a month. He's done a lot of this sort of work with me, but he's never done one on his own, see. He's almost graduated. So we can do you a deal. If James does the caesarean with me sitting over there telling him what to do, and if it lives, we'll charge you fifty dollars, plus mileage. And if it dies we'll just charge you the mileage for coming out here.'

Trevor thought about it for a minute. 'I don't really have anything to lose in that scenario, do I?'

'No, not really.'

'All right, we'll give it a go.'

'That's good. That's really good,' Bob said. 'Now if you can just piss off and leave us alone for the next hour or two that would be great. He doesn't need you looking over his shoulder worrying about what he's doing. You're a busy man you've got plenty to get on with.'

Trevor thanked us and went off to potter around in the machinery shed. Bob arranged a series of 44-gallon drums for me to use as instrument tables. He found a milk-crate-sized drum for himself to sit on. 'There's the cow, there's the drugs and there's the surgical instruments. You know what to do, so get going. Ask me when you need to ask me.' He pulled out a newspaper and started to read.

With the cow standing still in the crush, I opened up the rail on her left side, pulled out a scalpel and proceeded to use it like a cutthroat razor to shave a window about three inches wide by a foot long on the side of her. I prepped the skin with iodine to disinfect it. I put a local anaesthetic block into the gap between the vertebrae where I knew the nerves that felt pain down that whole flank operated. I poked her with a needle because I wanted to make sure she couldn't feel a thing. She didn't flinch. I moved the needle and checked another part.

'Stop poking the cow and get on with cutting it,' Bob piped up over the top of the *Inverell Times*. 'You know what you're doing. Hurry up.'

Here goes nothing. I sliced into the cow but nothing happened. So I sliced again, harder. They're made from leather, these cows. Much tougher than dogs and cats. I made my way into the abdomen where I found a lot of fluid from the internal infection that she was carrying. I probed around and pretty quickly got my hands on the uterus where I could feel the calf's back legs.

I grabbed the legs through the thickness of the uterus and picked up the whole lot and dragged it all over closer to the opening, bringing the legs inside the uterus up and out through the hole. We'd had it stressed upon us at uni that it was crucial to get that uterus out before opening it up.

I stabbed into the uterus, and all the fetid juices that had been stewing around the rotten carcass came welling up towards me. I cut along the uterus with my scissors, making a hole big enough for a calf to fit through, and then I let it fall down on the outside of the cow so the rest of the foul brew could drain away to the ground. If it had come out inside the cow it would have killed her. But something they hadn't bothered to teach us at uni was to stand clear. All this disgusting gunk splattered my boots and overalls.

'You're not coming in the car like that,' Bob called out. 'When you know what you're doing, you won't get that shit all over you. Look at you. You stink.'

I grabbed the back legs and pulled them out of the uterus. The calf came away fairly easily and hit the ground with a thud, a thick fog of disgusting odour coming with it and bouncing back up into my nostrils. I hooked out the decomposing placental material from the uterus and dropped that to the ground too. Bob came straight over and dragged it away, thankfully, because it smelled a terrible shade of horrendous. Experience had told him to wear a few pairs of gloves so he would be able to continue reading the paper afterwards.

'So now you've got to put it all back together,' he said.

My first job was to close the uterus and even though I'd tried to get everything out, there was no way I could get it completely clean, so future infection was almost a certainty.

'Make sure you close that properly,' Bob said, 'Otherwise she'll die and this will have all been a giant waste of everyone's time.'

There's a special suture pattern where you turn the uterus in on itself to make a watertight seal. I did that but wasn't certain it was going to seal, so I did another one over the top. I pushed it all back in and stitched up the muscle on her flank which is like sewing steak because that's exactly what I was doing – bringing two great chunks of beef together and stitching them through with great long needles. It had looked so neat and ordered when I'd cut my way through it an hour or so earlier, but after me rummaging around in there, it was like a traffic accident. The different layers of muscle were all over the place and I had no idea which bits were meant to connect with which. Still, I connected each bit to something, then stitched up the skin which was like mending a belt.

I was beat by this time but not as beat as the cow who'd stood there so calmly the whole time. I filled her with antibiotics and anti-inflammatories, then poured water into her stomach through a tube – providing her with hydration and electrolytes – to give her the best chance I could. I sprayed her with a lot of fly repellent too, because the fly season was coming and we didn't want them laying their eggs in her wound.

Bob called Trevor over and explained that he had to give her an antibiotic injection every day for at least the next week. Trevor looked pretty happy about it all. I felt happy, too, that I'd given this cow the best possible chance of survival. On the drive back Bob wasn't so happy about the smell I'd brought into the car on my boots, but I think he was pleased he'd been able to help a young bloke learn the job.

'You make sure you ring him tomorrow and find out how she's going. We've got to charge him if she makes it.'

So the next day I got into work on another of those frigid mornings. I went straight to the phone to ring Trevor but there was a message waiting for me on the desk: 'Trevor rang to say cow going well. Bright and happy and heaps better than yesterday.'

I phoned him a few days later and his voice was ecstatic. 'She's perfect. Couldn't be happier. Tell Bob to send me the bill.'

'I wouldn't be that confident she's still going to make it,' I said. 'Infection might get her yet.'

'You tell Bob I'll pay. She's lived long enough.'

When I told Bob this he turned to me, shaking his head. 'What an idiot. He should have just told us she died.'

You had to love Bob.

WHERE DID I COME FROM?

Anthony

All my peers were starting to panic, and I was inclined to join them. I was in my last rotation of the final year and I didn't have a job yet. A few of my better organised classmates had teed up positions and that just made the rest of us feel like we'd been left on the shelf.

So, with a week to go before graduation, I got my act into gear and put together a résumé. I'd once met a guy on a plane who owned a famous restaurant in Sydney called the Bathers' Pavilion. He told me that you should always apply for the job that you want, not the one that is being offered. So I took his advice and called all the well-respected mixed-animal practices in the Shoalhaven district on the NSW South Coast. I definitely wanted to go into mixed practice – working on big farm animals plus small family pets – and I loved the South Coast. Jobs were hard to come by in Sydney, but it was easier in the country, especially for guys. Country practices lean towards males because there's a perception that you need to be strong to do the job. There are plenty of smaller framed girls and guys who are fantastic large-animal vets, but the idea persists, particularly among farmers. There were only twenty-five males in our class of 130, and ten of those were overseas students. So there were only fifteen male vets looking for jobs in New

South Wales. Whether the perception was right or wrong, guys were in demand.

I phoned all the practices from Nowra to Kiama. When I called the clinic in the little town of Berry, the owners said they didn't have a job going but were happy for me to come in and meet them. Their names were Geoff and Geoff – Geoff Scarlett and Geoff Manning – and I knew of them by way of their reputation as the best cattle vets in the area.

When they took me into the tea room to have a chat, it was perplexing. The two Geoffs were starkly contrasting personalities. Geoff Manning stood a foot shorter than Geoff Scarlett and didn't have a lot to say. Geoff Scarlett, on the other hand, was very friendly and did all the talking. To add to my confusion, the head nurse, Jenny, was constantly interrupting from the doorway before eventually just sitting herself down to participate in proceedings. So while Geoff Scarlett conducted the interview that wasn't an interview, Geoff Manning seemed vaguely irritated that he had been disturbed from reading the *Herald* and Jenny couldn't contain her excitement that a new vet might be starting soon. She kept finishing Geoff Scarlett's sentences, saying things like, 'There is a great opportunity here for you, Anthony.'

I walked out thinking how weird they were. I jumped in my car and drove to Sydney, where a mate needed help digging a basement for his uncle's wine cellar. After an internship year with no paying job I needed the money. And at that stage it felt like digging holes might be my immediate future.

It was only a few days before the phone rang, however. I walked out from all the dust and noise of the basement into the full blast of a hot summer's day. Rushing to get my dust mask and ear protectors off while wiping my face with my cement-covered arm, I was finally able to take the call.

'Anthony, it's Geoff Scarlett from Berry here. Do you still want that job?'

'What job? There wasn't a job,' I said.

'Well, there is now,' he said. 'Are you interested?'

'Yes I am.'

This was a dream position with the top vets in an area I'd virtually grown up in. I was elated. Berry is a beautiful little town tucked in under the rugged escarpment, less than ten minutes' drive from the beach and only 20 minutes from our family farm. Geoff and I made plans for me to start in a few weeks' time and it was as simple as that. I got back on the shovel.

As it turned out, I received a couple more job offers. I was sorely tempted by one from Andrejs Medenis at Gerringong – a beautiful little town ten minutes from Berry, with deep-blue ocean to the east and deep-green dairy paddocks to the west. It truly was a magical spot to work in. And Andrejs was one of the reasons I had wanted to become a vet in the first place, because he was the vet for our farm at Foxground.

Both my parents were doctors. Dad was a radiologist and Mum was a GP. Though we lived in Sydney, Dad was a frustrated farmer. He'd spent his childhood holidays at the farms of his relations at Narromine and later at Gloucester, leaving him with a hankering for the country and some cattle. When I was seven, Mum and Dad bought eighty acres at Foxground, a little valley just west of Gerringong. It had been a deer farm, and deer need tall fences. One of my first memories of it was working with a pair of bolt cutters to help Dad cut down the tall chicken-wire fences and get the place ready to run cattle.

I used to love helping Dad. Wherever he was, I had to be. If he was working in the paddock, if he was on the tractor, whatever he was doing, I was there, boots on and ready to dig holes or mend fences. We did all our own work with the cows. We'd get Andrejs in for emergencies but Dad, Pa (my grandfather) and myself would do all the routine work like vaccinating, ear-tagging and marking. Pa was an old dairy farmer so he knew cattle.

For all that farm experience, I still had a lot to learn about how things actually worked. I was a very naïve child. I remember one afternoon when I was about ten, we'd been fencing and the sun was going down. Dad had just let the bull in with the cows and he was leaning on the gate watching the stud mingle with his harem. So I leaned on the gate and watched what the bull did too. The bull's name was Corby, he was a big poll Hereford with a wide chest and curly white hair on his forehead like a judge's wig. He was named after a boxer from the olden days named Gentleman Jim Corbett who was known to be a very fair fighter. But when I saw Corby enter the paddock with the cows he seemed anything but gentleman-like as he sniffed around their rear ends and then jumped up on the back of one with his long pink willy hanging out.

'What the hell is Corby doing Dad?' I asked in amazement.

Dad didn't answer with words. He looked at me like I was a freak, as if to say, 'Don't you know anything?'

'No, what's he doing?' I persisted.

'You know, he's making babies with the cow.'

'How?'

Dad kept looking at me strangely. I see now what a perfect opportunity this was for the big chat: father and son out there, just him and me, leaning on the gate, sun setting.

'Hasn't your mother explained to you what happens?'

I looked at him blankly.

'Rightio.' And he turned around and walked straight back to the house.

Where's Dad gone and what on earth is Corby doing to that cow?

Back home in Sydney a few days later I found a picture book on my bed called *Where Did I Come From?* I read it with great interest but still couldn't figure out why Dad hadn't just explained it to me out in the paddock. He didn't need the pictures. We had it occurring right there before our eyes.

Even though Dad was a doctor and we did a lot of the cattle work ourselves, sometimes he'd still need to get the vet out from Gerringong. As I said, the main one we saw was Andrejs, who seemed like a really nice man to me. Andrejs was tall with long blond hair. He was a surfie who'd grown up on the point at Werri Beach. He'd come out to the farm and the women would swoon. He had no shortage of assistants – often heavily made-up women in short skirts.

Andrejs's dad was also a vet. He'd started the practice in the 1950s. Back then, the NSW South Coast was such an unloved little backwater that they couldn't get vets to work there. Apparently there wasn't a single practitioner south of Wollongong. So the dairy co-operatives offered to rehome vets from Eastern Europe. The farmers got their vets and the vets escaped the poverty and injustice of post-war Europe.

Andrejs' dad, Arties 'Arty' Medenis, was one of the relocated vets. He started the Gerringong clinic and another vet, George Bouris, started the Berry practice.

Arty was still around then, but Andrejs did most of the work. I thought it looked like a very cool job. It was like the medical stuff I knew my parents did, but it was also outside and physical. For a kid, that was very appealing. So the seed of my career was planted then by Andrejs; and now here he was offering me a job almost twenty years later.

As difficult as the decision was, it made more sense to go to Berry. Arty still owned the Gerringong practice, and even though Andrejs was going to take it over it was always going to remain Arty's practice with Arty's rules while ever he was around. Arty had never taken a partner in more than fifty years of practice, despite much cajoling. So it seemed that there was less opportunity for advancement there.

The Geoffs at Berry, on the other hand, were well into their careers, perhaps nearing the end of their working lives. The words of Jenny, the vet nurse, kept coming to mind too. It seemed there would be a good opportunity for me to set down roots in Berry.

George Bouris had sold the Berry clinic to Geoff Manning about thirty years earlier, but people were still talking about him. I heard stories about how he was very proud of his physique, yet he'd always have a cigarette in his mouth, no matter how disgusting the job at hand was. He might be pulling out a rotten placenta, but the cigarette would be there dangling and smouldering. And during calvings, he'd strip down to his undies – leopard-skin briefs – and strut around, dominating the cow with his sheer presence.

Old dairy man Bruce McIntosh told me how one day he'd said to George he should go easy on the smokes, that they'd kill him eventually.

'Look at me. I am a bull. Nothing can kill me,' he'd proclaimed.

A few years later he was in hospital with throat cancer. In his mind it was just a minor ailment and he'd be back at work in weeks, so instead of selling the practice he signed an agreement to go into partnership with Geoff Manning. A few days later he was dead.

So Geoff came down facing a career of hard yakka working for dairy farmers. He built the practice up, brought Geoff Scarlett in a couple of years later, and then they expanded the small-animal side of things in partnership over close to thirty years. In that time the area changed massively. Even when I was a kid, nobody wanted to go to Berry. The Southern Highlands was where all the money went; and the masses, if they went south at all, went to the beaches.

But it started changing with a French restaurant in the 1970s, then an antique shop, and off it went, so that by the time I moved down full time to work, the main street was awash with homewares, nick-nacks, cafés and restaurants. And there were far fewer dairy cows; instead there were horses, alpacas and Chihuahuas called Robert.

I remember driving down to start work. Coming out of Sydney it's all freeway and eucalypts and semi-urban sprawl. But then you skirt the folds of a small mountain on which lush green cow paddocks slope down to the breakers – the glorious Kiama bends. Coming out of the last bend, you see the greenness dotted with cabbage-tree palms stretching out in front, and you get a waft of cow manure and grass and ocean breeze. You try to catch a sneaky look at the surf to see what the waves are like but you're doing eighty down a tricky slope so you can't look long enough to tell. But it's those barnyard smells along with the ocean and the scent of the different flowers blooming then – be they dandelion or fireweed – that all go into the great big perfume mixer and hit you like a climate-controlled door. I would come to see this place as my gateway to home.

I moved into Dad's new farm near Nowra. Since I wasn't taking the Gerringong job, I rang my university mate, Matt Izzo, one of the NROC veterans, to let him know about it.

'Do you want a job and a place to live rent free?'

'Sounds too good to pass up.' So he took the Gerringong job and moved in with me at Depot Farm, a magical place nestled into the sheer cliffs that drop to the Shoalhaven River west of Nowra.

Dad had forty-five head of Angus cattle on the place and it was calving season. Early on in my stay, I heard a cow bellowing a really long, loud honk before I went to sleep. She woke me before dawn, still going loud and strong. It was different to a normal bellow, and she was obviously distressed – that noise transcends language. I thought I'd better go and investigate, so I pulled on a thick jacket, beanie and boots and followed the honking across the uneven paddocks until I saw the cow's black shape down at the far end of the block. She was standing at the top of an embankment that dropped to the river 20 metres below. As the first grey streaks of light started to crack the sky, I looked down the steep bank over the mud and wombat holes and tree roots and, sure enough, there was her calf at the water's edge. *Shivers!* The calf was pacing backwards and forwards on a narrow muddy part of the riverbed, bellowing for its mother. I knew that the water would come in a long way at high tide, so the calf was going to be in serious trouble.

When I'd got up, I'd dressed for work at the clinic figuring that since I was up I might as well pop in early. I knew if I went down to get that calf I was going to end up a mess. So I took off my clothes, hanging my jacket, shirt and trousers from a nearby tree. When I stepped out of my boots, my toes were in instant agony from the freezing ground. In just my undies, which, disappointingly, were not leopard skin, I climbed down the bank towards this little black calf that looked about three weeks old. At that age, calves are no longer teetering cute little balls of helplessness. Their muscles are already filling out and they run like greyhounds. I tried to corner him, but he was not in a frame of mind to be cooperative, so I had to tackle him. The little guy just went berserk. He thrashed and bellowed, while Mum, up above, increased her decibels to the point where I started expecting a noise complaint from the neighbours. Somehow I managed to lift the forty-odd kilo calf up the first part of the bank. I then had to hold it down while trying to climb up myself, before lifting the writhing body again and trying to get it up to the next level of the bank. I repeated this process a few times, but eventually I was absolutely exhausted. And so was the calf.

I just lay on top of it and looked at it. It looked at me. I'm surprised it didn't laugh. I was covered in red clay that barely concealed my goose bumps and blue feet.

'I can't get you up any further, mate. I need help.'

I let the calf go, climbed up the bank and ran back to get Izzo. Still in my undies and, covered in mud, I couldn't go in the house, so I knocked hard. Izzo came to the door: 'Anthony, I know you're into your fitness, but this is ridiculous.'

'Mate, you're about to look the same,' I said.

I told him the story and he didn't need any convincing. Gotta love Izzo, he's mad. Before I knew it he'd stripped down to his undies and one white body in blue undies and one red Claymation figure were streaking across the paddock, back to the scene of the action. It was NROC reassembled.

With the two of us and a length of rope, it was pretty easy getting the calf up and we came back to shower and get ready for work. Even though I'd turned the hot tap right down, it scalded my frosted skin. I had clay everywhere, but I couldn't stay in the shower long because I had to get ready for work again. And I was on call, so I might be required at any minute.

As I was about to head out the door I heard the home phone ringing. This was odd because the only people with the number were Dad and Pa and neither of them would call so early. I doubled back and grabbed the receiver off the old yellow dial-up phone, curious to hear who it was.

A wolf whistle came down the line loud enough to rupture an eardrum. 'Looking good boys!' It was one of our two female neighbours. They were just cacking themselves.

They hung up and almost immediately my mobile rang. 'It's Peter Walsh from Kangaroo Valley here.' He spoke in the steady tones of those who live by the rhythms of the land. I've since heard it said that the Walshes had been in Kangaroo Valley so long Noah dropped them off the Ark on the way past. 'I've got a calving here and I think it's bad,' Peter said.

I have since come to learn that because the Walshes are such experienced cattle people, if you are called to their dairy for a calving, it's going to be a bad one, because if it was easy they would have got it out themselves. But I knew none of this then. I was only new to the job. I grasped enough, however, to sense that the Walshes were big clients whom I would have to attend to diligently. With red clay still under my fingernails, I jumped in the car to drive over the mountain to Kangaroo Valley.

I pulled up at the house in my old Magna. Peter, tall, greying and wiry, came over to greet me wearing the standard dairy farmer's uniform of black gumboots and a faded blue flannelette shirt. 'She's just over here,' he said, pointing with his great ham-like hands to a ramshackle old yard and a crush that looked like it too had been dropped overboard from the Ark. The cow was in there, but the part that would normally close onto her neck to hold her firm was wide open because it didn't work. Nor did the gate that usually closes behind the cow to stop her kicking you. So the only way we could keep this cow in the crush was to wedge a bit of wood in behind her, pushing the animal so far forwards that her head was pressed into the front of the crush. It was less than ideal.

Peter saw my look of concern. 'We've got our main yards over at the dairy down the road, but we keep the cows that are about to calve up here at the house so we can keep an eye on them.'

I dipped my hands in iodine and lubricant and went in to have a feel around. Even with my limited experience I knew the cervix had dilated, but the calf had spun 90 degrees in the abdomen so the uterus had twisted. Imagine twisting a partially inflated balloon and you get the picture of how this calf's exit route had been closed off.

I also knew that a caesarean was the only hope of saving mother and baby. I was lucky that my second-last rotation as a student had been at Finley in the Riverina, near the Victorian border, where there are a lot of irrigated dairy farms. I had a great rotation there with vets named Petso and Butch, and ended up doing quite a few surgeries – calvings, twisted stomachs and caesareans. I'd done a couple of caesareans alone, observed a few others and assisted with a few more, so I felt pretty comfortable with the whole thing.

Because I was so new, one of the Geoffs would be nominated as my backup when I was on call, so that if there was something I couldn't handle, they were there to come and help. But up at Kangaroo Valley, I was out of mobile range. I could have asked the Walshes to call from their house; however, I felt I could handle it and I really wanted to prove that.

There were two big complicating factors. One was that the Walshes breed big, big animals. Holsteins are already one of the tallest breeds of cow in the world and the Walshes seemed intent on making theirs even larger. My head was in line with this cow's withers (the bumps at the top of the shoulder blades). The other complication was that to do a caesarean you need access to the cow's left side. But the left side of this crush didn't open, only the right. Normally the cow's head would be contained in the crush and you'd swing the left rail out to perform the operation; however, that option wasn't available to us. Peter quietly mentioned that Geoff (Manning) would normally reverse the cow into the crush, tie her head to the rail with a halter and then tie her body into the crush with a piece of rope.

This was going to be a doozy.

Peter put a halter on the cow and then tied a rope from the head bale back around her body to pin it in there. It looked okay, but I knew that if she became agitated such a big animal could thrash her way free with ease. And at that time we didn't use many sedatives. The only one we had, xylazine, was dangerous in cattle. They are super sensitive to it, so if you give them too much, they go down. The last thing you want when you are doing a caesarean is for the cow to suddenly want to lie down. All the weight of the abdomen on the ground pushes the guts up and they all come out through the hole you've created or, worse, the cow flops onto the hole and you can't access the calf any more.

So I put in the local anaesthetic and confidently cut into the cow's left side. A cow's rumen, the largest of the four stomachs, sits on the left. If you make your cut on the right, all the guts fall out, but, if you do it on the left, the rumen is large enough to act as a plug. If you cut too deep, however, you will lacerate the rumen and the cow's abdomen will fill with grass and bacteria and that will be the end of her.

I could see the light pink, spongy mass of the rumen pushing up against the hole, so I knew that hadn't happened. I could also see the shape of the calf in the uterus, luckily very close to the cut. I manoeuvred one of the calf's legs out through my incision. I was then able to cut into the uterus, allowing a shower of contaminated tea-coloured amniotic fluid to pour out onto the ground and all over me. Saturated twice in the one day and it wasn't even seven o'clock yet.

Things started to improve from there and I was able to reach into the cow's uterus to locate the calf's other front leg and head. Peter looped straps over the calf's feet and with an almighty heave we delivered the calf through the cow's flank.

It was alive and female. Godly clouds form over you in these moments, accompanied by swelling violins and shafts of light. The farmer is elated because a female is ultimately worth thousands of dollars while a male calf is almost worthless. The vet is elated because both lives have been saved and the client is happy.

But there was still work to do. Peter held the uterus for me with his massive gnarled hands while I stitched it up with a watertight suture pattern. After that, it was straightforward to untwist the uterus now that it was empty. Everything went beautifully with this enormous animal, which, at any moment could have had a conniption, snapped those ropes and landed on top of me.

Peter hadn't said much during the process, but the mere fact he'd let me have a go was praise enough. When he shook my hand and slapped my back on the way out, I knew he was happy.

I was very chuffed with myself as I got back into the Magna, covered with placenta and dirt, to drive back to Berry. I wound back up the hill through the rainforest, past a big wombat and a scurrying lyrebird. This truly was a magic day. *They'll all be suitably impressed when I tell them about my morning.* Topping the rise at Woodhill Mountain brought me back into mobile range and no sooner had the Magna started the descent into Berry than the phone rang.

'Where are you?' It was Geoff Scarlett and he was angry. 'You were meant to start work an hour ago.'

'I'm on the way back from Kangaroo Valley.'

'What are you doing?'

'I got a call from the Walshes. I had to do a caesarean. I'm on my way back.'

'Oh, okay. You need to do a caesarean. I'm on my way.'

'No, Geoff, I've done it. I'm on my way back.'

'What do you mean, you've done it?'

'I did it myself. I'll be back in Berry in fifteen.'

'Why the hell didn't you call me?'

'I was out of range and I didn't think I needed help. I'm happy to do them on my own.'

I think the two Geoffs were a bit taken aback. At uni our year was the very first to do an entire year of prac work before being let loose on the world. All the new vets they'd ever seen before had only done six weeks.

I got back in and they were still a bit shocked and cranky that I hadn't called. 'It was a nice black and white heifer,' I said, 'and the mother looks like she'll be fine.'

'Okay,' said Geoff, 'but what's that red gunk coming out your ear?'

'Oh that. That's another story.'

ALL PIGS GREAT ...

James

As uni drew to a close and everyone's attention turned to what they were going to do next, I started to think about putting a CV together. Before I did anything, I figured I'd better call the Inverell and Barraba clinics for references. That turned out to be a good time-saver because instead of writing a reference, both of them offered me a job.

It was a big decision to make. Whichever one I chose, it was going to affect the rest of my life, so I didn't want to get it wrong. I am terrible at making decisions. I overthink everything. If I have a problem, I go from the worst possible outcome and work my way backwards to the best. Until such time as I have thought through every single permutation of what could happen, I can't sleep. It might be 3 a.m. before I decide I can switch off.

I had loved working with Bob at Inverell and with Ben at Barraba. The mix of smallies and largies was similar at the two clinics, but I knew Bob had a tightly managed structure at Inverell, while I was likely to be cut loose a little bit more at Barraba. Barraba Veterinary Clinic had an excellent reputation with graduates and, as far as I could tell, they were all still on good terms, so that was a positive sign. On top of that, Barraba was two hours closer to Sydney, where my girlfriend lived. Such things matter when you're twenty-three.

So I went for Barraba. And if it was responsibility I was seeking, I got it. On my second day there, Ben called me over. 'Well James,' he said. 'You did a month's prac work here. You kind of know where everything is and how things work, so you can handle the branch clinic at Manilla on your own today. Good luck. Call me if you need me.'

The fear must have shown in my face. He adopted a very soothing tone. 'Don't worry. You know more than you think you know. You're better than you think you are. Just get out there and do it.'

So that's what I did. I jumped in the car and drove the 45 kilometres south to Manilla and waited for things to go wrong. I spent that first day in abject terror that something complicated would come through the door or, worse, that I'd stuff up something simple and make it complicated.

Fortunately for me, Manilla Veterinary Clinic was staffed by an amazing nurse. Suzanne Barton was a bubbly, enthusiastic Englishwoman in her late thirties. She'd come to Australia on a working holiday and when she was due to go home, a badly broken leg intervened. She ended up getting married and making her life here. Eventually, most of her family had followed her out. Without Suzanne I'm pretty sure I wouldn't have survived those early days. We became good friends. Her kids would get dropped off at the clinic by the school bus and would kick around in the afternoon, so I got dragged into the orbit of the family.

Later that first day, Jessica Taylor, a slightly built redhead came into the clinic and chatted to Suzanne before walking towards me. 'G'day James, I'm Jessica. Welcome to Manilla. We play touch on Wednesdays. So, ah, yeah, you'll be playing?' It wasn't really a question.

'Ah, okay.'

'Good. After the game you'll come back to our place for dinner. I'll cook one week, you cook the other. So we'll see you Wednesday.' My predecessor, Tim, had played, so I had no choice. That was how everyone seemed to treat me. I loved the feeling of being involved and being thrown straight into the mix of what was happening. And I still owe Jessica and her husband, Paul, quite a few dinners.

I handled everything the animal kingdom threw at me on that first day and I started to allow myself to think that maybe Ben had been right when he had talked about me being better than I thought I was.

On my second day at Manilla, he dropped in to see how I was going and we were chatting away when Suzanne came in with a call to go out to a property to euthanase a dog and a pig.

Ben quickly ran through his preferred technique for putting dogs to sleep. 'Now, with the pig, it's very straightforward: you go through the ear vein. You'll see the big vein. Just put it in there. You'll have to guess the pig's weight to figure out the dosage.'

I must have looked unconvinced. My knowledge of pigs was probably less than sound. In our crucial fourth year at uni, the pig lecturer had left suddenly, so they had had to get in a replacement, and all his instruction was compressed into one big porcine week. Unfortunately, I had missed pretty much that entire week. It just happened to be the week before *Barbie Grog*, the vet revue. Anthony and I, plus a bunch of others, were on the organising committee. We took our responsibilities very seriously and dedicated a lot of time to them. It was a matter of inter-year pride to put on a good show. On top of that, I was still trying to hold down a part-time job and so my pig-lecture attendance was poor to say the least. Our contribution to the revue – titled 'Blinding Nemo' – went down a treat. Unfortunately, that didn't translate into marks.

With the pig test looming on Monday morning, I'd had to work at the call centre on Sunday afternoon in Sydney. I got back to Camden at 9 p.m. and opened the pig text book. It was stiff and clean smelling because its pages had never before been turned. I started reading it that night and asked a few questions of one of our more diligent mates who explained some things to me about the peculiarities of the pig's digestive tract. I continued reading the book into the quiet hours, long after everyone else's lights went out. I finished the last page at 4 a.m., got up at 7 a.m., put on my cross-dressing outfit – into which I'd put more time than I had my studies – stumbled into the exam in my ill-fitting heels, found the test pretty easy with all that fresh info bubbling through my brain, got a distinction, and hardly retained a single piece of pig knowledge.

This all flashed through my mind as I stood there wondering how I was going to put this pig to sleep, and perhaps Ben recognised something in my expression – a peculiar mix of grimace and grin.

'It's all right,' he said. 'I'll come with you. I'll come with you.'

Ben was an incredibly bubbly, energetic kind of guy. He said everything in short, sharp sentences, often repeating the conclusion of the sentence. 'Do this. Do this.' It was almost a mumble. He had a head full of knowledge, but his brilliant mind went too fast for his mouth to keep up, so the words often came out as a deep rumble and sentences merged into each other. You'd look at him, wondering what on earth he was talking about, and there were plenty of conversations that left me slightly more confused than when I started. He did everything at pace. He lived opposite the Barraba clinic and he'd drive across the road at high speed, pull up and say, 'Ah crikey! Forgot my bag. Forgot my bag.' Then he'd turn around, run back to his house then back to the clinic. There was no walking. We called him The Big Red Chief.

So we drove out to the property like we had a siren on the roof. That was good, as it gave me less time to ponder my shortcomings. At least this job wasn't going to require any deep understanding of porcine biology. We just had to insert a needle, after all. And I actually knew a little bit about killing pigs. Our university rotations included piggeries, where you were exposed to the brutal nature of intensive pig production, and I had assisted in the euthanasia of many unfortunate piglets.

This, however, wasn't a piglet.

A lovely middle-aged couple, Joan and John, came out to greet us. Their 1200-acre farm in normally fertile country was turning to red dust as a mid-summer dry spell took hold. They led us into a shed close to the house. It looked like it was intended for vehicles but was mainly being used for the storage of corrugated iron, old fridges and bookshelves.

'Fred's over here,' said John, clearly upset, guiding us to a large kelpie cross lying on a mattress by a wall. Fred looked old and tired and didn't bother shifting from his bed as we approached. He examined us with forlorn eyes that appeared to say it was time to go to doggie heaven, but as Ben reached down to touch him he bared his teeth and emitted a savage, low growl that told us maybe he wasn't so ready.

'Mmmmm,' said Ben. 'Mmmmm. Didn't bring a muzzle. No muzzle. Mmmmmm. Mmmmmm. James, you hold the dog. I'll inject the vein.' Fred had been urinating on himself because he hadn't been able to get up off the bed. So he wasn't going to get up to bite me, but each time I reached towards him, he showed me those broken yellow fangs.

I grabbed his stinking yellow mattress and put it over the top of him as his teeth bit hard into the old foam. That allowed us to pull a front leg out and Ben managed to get the needle in.

'Thank you so much,' Joan said, through gentle sobs, as Fred drifted off. 'Sorry he was so difficult. He's not normally like that. But it was nice and peaceful in the end.'

'Yes, it was very sad,' Ben said. 'But he'd definitely reached the end. You made the right decision.'

'We'd better go and do the pig now,' John said. He had the air of a man who knows he's got to keep busy lest he show any more emotion.

'What's wrong with the pig?' Ben asked in a more farmerly voice.

'Well Winston's eleven months old. We got him as an orphan and we fed him … and we, ah, fed him a lot. Winston's gotten so big his joints are collapsing under his weight. He's got some sort of early arthritis. He's just too big.'

They took us around the back of the farm buildings and Joan banged on a food tin. At first nothing happened, but then off in the distance I made out a swirl of red dust with a great pink mass in the middle of it, lurching and heaving towards us in a half-run, half-stagger kind of motion.

As it got closer, I realised it was the biggest pig I'd ever seen: a white landrace with huge testicles hanging out the back and huge tusks at the front. The hint of food had made Winston forget the pain in his joints but, with no food to be had, he began to hobble like a cripple as he came to inspect us. I realised Winston was also the friendliest pig I'd ever seen in my very limited experience. He wanted to be pals.

'Okay, I can see what you're talking about with his size and his joints,' Ben said. 'We could try to get him better. Put him on a diet and give him some medications. Yes, a diet and medications.'

'No, he's too difficult for us to handle,' Joan said. 'He keeps breaking out. We've tried fixing him up, but we've reached a point where we just can't do any more.'

'Have you thought about sending him off to the abattoir?' Ben asked.

'We couldn't do that,' John said. 'We couldn't eat Winston.'

'Okay,' Ben said, turning to me. 'You hold Winston and I'll inject him.'

'No problem.'

Joan brought a bucket of food out and Winston tucked in with squeals of delight, as if never before had such exquisite pig pellets graced the plate of man or beast. I took hold of Winston's flapping pink ear, trying to hold him steady. But between each mouthful of his most excellent pellets he flicked his head around to check out the visitors and the action, knocking me – all of 65 kilograms – around like I wasn't there.

Ben couldn't get the needle anywhere near the vein. 'Has he ever had a snout rope?' Ben asked.

'No. We tried once, but he went ballistic,' Joan said.

Ben and I swapped places. He tried to use his greater weight while I took the syringe filled with the lethal green barbiturate anaesthetic Lethabarb – commonly known as Nembutal. But it didn't make any difference. We must have spent fifteen minutes trying different ways to restrain the pig, but Winston could not be contained. We attempted sedating him with injections into his muscles but he wouldn't cooperate and the injections were only going into the enormous rolls of body fat instead of his bloodstream. They had no effect.

Eventually, Ben broke off and went over to Joan and John. 'Look, we can't inject the pig, so a clear gunshot to the head may be a humane solution.'

'Yeah, we understand. That's okay,' said John. 'We realise it's our fault that we've never handled the pig before. We have no facilities.' So John went away to get the gun.

'Yes, yes,' murmured Ben. 'This will be much easier. Much easier. We'll shoot the pig. Definitely shoot the pig.'

Ben's from a practical farming background and has had to use guns to euthanase animals many times before. He's a brilliant surgeon and a great vet, and one of the most pragmatic people I've ever come across. But his thinking was so ingrained with pragmatism that I suspect he sometimes struggled to understand how emotional some of our clients could be in their decision making. His outlook on life was obviously much treasured by our clients, as he was not only respected in the profession but was seen as part of the furniture by the local communities.

John came back with a .22. I looked at it doubtfully. *That's not gunna work.* Though I could remember little about pigs, I did know that they have a very thick, bony casing on the front of their skull so that they can attack things with their heads. This makes it very difficult to shoot a pig in the cranium.

Ben looked at the gun in much the same way as I had, but then he seemed to start convincing himself that the task was possible. 'He's only eleven months old, so his bony plates won't have properly fused yet. Yes, this gun should do the trick. Yep, it'll do the trick if fired at the right spot.'

Ben was one of the most respected vets in Australia. Who was I to argue?

We put some more food in the trough, and Joan and John retired to the other side of the open-fronted shed.

'Have you shot him yet?' one of them asked. Ben and I looked at each other, not quite believing the question. These were solid country folk, but emotions were obviously playing on their faculties.

'No, you'll hear the gunshot when we do,' I called back.

Eventually, Winston stopped snorting and sniffing and doing all that pig stuff long enough to present a target. Ben lined him up and was just about to fire when Winston suddenly twigged to what was happening. He ran like a racehorse to the far side of the paddock, his arthritis remarkably improved at the sight of the .22.

Winston was gone, along with our chances of finishing the job. I heard a rattling noise and saw Joan advancing onto the edge of the paddock with the food tin. Winston pulled up in his tracks like a showjumper refusing to take a hurdle. He turned around and proceeded to trot back towards us as though nothing had ever happened.

'How did he know?' I asked, but Ben wasn't listening. I could see his mind churning at high speed.

'Okay, looks like the gun's not going to work, so here's what we'll do. We're going to inject him in the testicles with Lethabarb. It's what some vets did when they were castrating pigs in the old days before we had good anaesthetics. They'd inject the pig there, it would fall asleep, we'd cut out the testicle with the Lethabarb in it, and then the pig would wake up.'

Ben suggested I should hold the pig still. But once again I contributed almost nothing to the process. Ben snuck up behind Winston and jammed Lethabarb into his testicles. Once again, Winston shrieked and ran like a racehorse to the far side of the paddock, but Joan shook the tin and he turned around and came trotting straight back. She filled the bucket again and Winston pigged out blissfully. We'd almost shot him. We'd stabbed him in the testicles. We'd given him two buckets of food. And he was still hungry. No wonder his joints were collapsing.

The Lethabarb took about ten minutes to kick in, then Winston started to look woozy.

'Right, James, see if you can hold his ear now. I reckon you can get that ear now.'

And I could. Ben came in with the big green syringe, put the Lethabarb into the vein and Winston promptly passed away. In doing so, however, he fell onto Ben, wedging him with his giant pink corpse against the corrugated-iron wall of the shed.

John, Joan and I contemplated getting the tractor to drag Winston off, but we managed to shift enough of the pink ripples of fat and meat for Ben to pull himself free and climb over the body.

'Yes, well, he appears to be dead,' Ben said.

The owners were once again very thankful for our efforts but we didn't make much eye contact with them as we picked up our gear and headed for the car.

'Okay, we'll be off then. We've got a lot of work backing up at the clinic.' Which was true. We'd been gone for hours on this five-minute job.

We drove in absolute silence to the front gate. I got out to open it. Ben drove through. I shut it behind him and got back in. He was sitting there looking blankly at the steering wheel. He put the car into gear, but didn't move forwards.

'Let us never speak of this again,' he said. And off we drove. Slowly.

... AND SMALL

Anthony

When you're a new vet, you get the quirky jobs. If a call comes in for a macaw or a hermit crab, the senior partners take off like ducks in hunting season. And so it was when Geoff Scarlett handed me the phone one day: 'Here's one for your run to the Heads.'

There was a woman on the line with a warm voice. 'Hello love, I was hoping you could drop some Baytril off for our guinea pig. He's got a bladder complaint.'

Being a diligent young vet, I felt the need to set her straight. 'I can't just sell you antibiotics. We're not a pharmacy. I need to come out and examine the guinea pig first.'

I was expecting my suggestion to meet with resistance. People think you're trying to overservice them. Or at least they think they know better and that all they need is the antibiotic and they'll be on their way. But to my surprise it wasn't like that at all.

'That would be great,' she said. 'How soon can you come?'

The caller lived in the quiet seaside village of Shoalhaven Heads, about ten minutes' drive from Berry. I did a run of house calls out there every Tuesday afternoon. So I made the appointment for early in the run. It was two sisters who lived in a flat little house on Oval Drive.

It had almost no front yard, but what they did have was manicured. I walked through the front door into the living room and there on the floor were a fluffy white rabbit and a brown guinea pig with a striking black stripe. The animals appeared to live a harmonious life, grazing grass and pellets off the carpet. The house was surprisingly clean, all things considered, and I noted the animals had a designated toileting zone on newspapers, which they appeared to frequent. They weren't at all startled by my entry, and when I sat on the floral-patterned lounge, the big fluffy rabbit hopped over, seeking attention like a cat or a dog.

I examined the guinea pig, whose name was Byron, and saw a lot of urine staining and scalding around his penis – a clear indication of urinary-tract infection.

The sisters, Myra and Val Hawken, explained that they'd just moved down from the western suburbs of Sydney. Byron's problem had been around for years, but their old vet never seemed to pay it much attention. He'd prescribe the Baytril and the problem would go away, but within a month or so it always came back.

Myra and Val weren't that old, but their clothes and buckle-up shoes seemed in keeping with their names – conservative and from a bygone era.

I explained again about not being a pharmacist and that we were obliged to examine animals before we could prescribe antibiotics. I explained that Baytril is an antibiotic that is safe to give to most 'exotic pets'. (We use this term for any animal that is not a cat, a dog or a farm animal, though it frustrates most exotic-animal vets, as creatures like guinea pigs are hardly exotic.) A lot of vets will give an injection of Baytril and prescribe a bottle for take-home use simply to be seen to be doing something. Arties Medenis always said that you needed to give an injection, even if it was water, otherwise the client would think that you were not trying.

That's what Myra and Val were expecting here, but instead they got me. They must have thought I was being a presumptuous smarty pants, trying to rip them off with all manner of expensive tests when all they wanted was the Baytril. But I pushed on. 'I'll give you the antibiotics this time around because it seems correct and you've had that treatment in the past, but if the infection comes back again, I think we have to draw a line in the sand and investigate.'

'Well, we think that's a really good idea,' said Myra with a good deal of enthusiasm. 'Let's do that. Frankly, we're getting sick of the whole cycle.'

I was shocked.

'We'll give you a call if it comes back,' Val said.

I left and went about my rounds, not giving Byron any more thought until a couple of weeks later when Myra called on a Saturday morning. 'It's the guinea pig,' she said. 'We think the infection's come back. Can we bring him in for you to have a look at?'

'Of course,' I said. 'We're free now.' They were at the clinic within the hour.

Val explained that the Baytril had worked for a time but the infection was back now, probably worse than ever. I pulled Byron out of his cage and put him on the stainless steel table. The skin around his groin and back legs was stained dark brown. He stank and blisters were forming where the ever-present urine was scalding his skin.

'He's really miserable at home and he's barely eating. He doesn't like attention any more. It's like he just wants to wallow in his own misery,' Val said.

'Where do we go to from here?' Myra asked. Good question. I realised I had no idea. I'd been saying we couldn't just keep on doling out antibiotics, but the truth was that I had no concept of what else we should do. I had to think fast. *If this was a cat or a dog, what would you do?*

'Okay, we need to collect a urine sample,' I said, full of authority and confidence. 'And we need an X-ray.'

'What is an X-ray going to achieve?' Myra asked politely.

Gulp. 'Ummm. It's going to rule out a tumour or a cancer,' I said with calm self-assurance. 'And we have to make sure he doesn't have anything that predisposes him to this condition.'

'How much will that cost?' Val asked.

We'd been going well but I expected to lose them now. 'It'll be about $150 for the X-ray and $25 for the urine test.'

'Okay, good. Let's do it.'

I took Byron out the back to admit him into hospital, along with his overnight bag containing grass, blankets, fluffy toys and pellets. This was one very loved guinea pig.

Geoff and Geoff were back there. 'What have you got in the box?' asked Geoff Scarlett.

'A guinea pig.' I saw their eyebrows rise up, and perhaps the hint of an eye roll.

'Right, and what's wrong with it?'

I explained the situation to Geoff and his face slowly fell. 'We have never X-rayed a guinea pig before. Do the clients know how much this is all going to cost?'

'Yep.'

'Well, I guess we can give it a go.' So with my bosses looking on, somewhat bemused, I collected urine and ultrasounded Byron. He was a very cooperative patient, but he didn't like being jabbed and having the cold ultrasound probe pressed into his side. Through all the wriggling I noticed a funny shadow in the bladder wall. I did an X-ray to get a better look. At least with an X-ray all Byron had to do was sit there.

I had to figure out how to set the factors for the X-ray, a complicated task like manually setting an SLR camera. Given that no one had ever imaged a guinea pig at Berry before, we didn't know what factors to use, but I managed to get a clear shot. When the image came out, my mouth dropped. There was an enormous white blob sitting in Byron's bladder, obviously a bladder stone. It was highly likely that this was what was causing Byron's problems. A bladder stone builds up from a tiny particle, layer by layer, like an oyster, and if there are bacteria in the bladder when the layer is forming, the bacteria will be trapped in that layer. So it becomes a big irritable ball of infection. If it dissolves a bit, the infection is unleashed.

I was pretty pleased with myself for getting to the bottom of it. Byron was the first guinea pig to have ever received that level of investigation at Berry vet clinic. On the other hand, this meant that we would have to embark on a surgery that none of us had ever done before, and that was a pretty intimidating thought, especially given Byron's privileged position in the Hawken household.

I eventually summoned up the courage to call Val. I headed outside so that I could talk privately on my mobile. Sure enough, as soon as I got hold of Val, Jenny felt it necessary to hang out a basket of washing. There was no privacy and no hiding out the back.

I explained to Val that the stone was like having a pebble in your shoe, it was moving around and irritating the lining of Byron's bladder.

'Okay then, what are we going to do about it?' she asked. I could tell that the two of them were trying to squeeze in to listen to the one phone.

I didn't have a plan but I winged it, thinking of Byron as if he were a cat. 'We'll have to remove the stone,' I said. 'And that's going to require surgery.'

'Oh, dear. All right. Let's do that then. Call us when you've done it.' And that was that. They didn't even give me the opportunity to recommend referral to a specialist. I could feel myself getting further in over my head, knowing that the Geoffs knew as much about guinea-pig surgery as I did.

This was my first experience of dealing with people who were pursuing treatment of animals that we wouldn't normally consider to be of high value. Since then I've seen it all the time and it's becoming increasingly common. Reptiles and small hindgut fermenters like guinea pigs are becoming more common as pets as backyards shrink. The veterinary profession has to move with it. A hundred years ago, horses provided the majority of vet work. With the rise of the motor car, that fell away and there was an increase in vet calls for cattle and sheep, but people seldom treated cats and dogs. That all changed after World War II and then we began to see this further shift towards smaller animals. An animal's value was no longer simply as a productive asset, but as a friend and a companion. People loved their pets, and wanted to help them. And that's why we were about to do a $350 surgery on a $7 guinea pig.

So I embarked on a surgical journey.

I went straight to our thick volumes of conference proceedings, those dusty great books with yellowy blue covers. On the spines, they had the topics of papers that had been delivered at various conferences. It was still in the early days of the internet so there wasn't much online at that time. I hunted through the volumes until I found one on pocket pets. I rustled through pages that looked like they'd been typed on a typewriter and I found an item on surgery for guinea pigs. Eureka! I quickly read through the article, trying to glean what I could, but the only relevant line seemed to be: 'Be careful not to kill the guinea pig with the anaesthetic.' Thanks for that, I thought.

Next I called a specialist, Dr Tom Donnelly, in Sydney who focused on exotics and he talked me through my options.

He stressed that indeed the most difficult part of operating on these small pets is managing the anaesthetic because they've got a very high metabolic rate. They metabolise the anaesthetic very quickly, so you need to use a lot. And they've got a large surface area relative to body size, so they get cold very quickly – in fact, you can kill them with cold during the procedure. 'They also have bizarre and difficult-to-navigate airways, so trying to get a tube in is difficult,' Tom said. 'Apart from that it's not different from doing the procedure in a cat – midline approach, find the bladder, open it, get the stones out and stitch it up with a watertight pattern. Don't starve the guinea pig at any point. Anaesthetise it with grass in its mouth and wake it up with access to grass or pellets because with its high metabolism it needs to eat constantly.' At the end of the conversation Tom reiterated what I'd already figured: 'Don't kill the guinea pig with anaesthetic.' And with that he was gone.

Feeling as ready as I was ever going to be, I enlisted Geoff Scarlett as my anaesthetist and also for reassurance. We knocked Byron out by placing a small cat mask over his face, flooding the mask with oxygen and what seemed like an enormous volume of anaesthetic gas. Once he was asleep, I was able to pass a tiny tube down his throat and into his lungs. The tube would serve to maintain a clear airway and provide continued anaesthetic gas to keep him asleep. We moved Byron into the sterile surgery and lay him on his back. Jenny clipped the bristly hair off his abdomen and did her best to clean the area of rank urine and bacteria. We covered his entire body with a large sterile green surgery drape that had a tiny operating hole in it. The idea of the drape is to provide access to the area of interest and cover everything else. It all looked a little ridiculous. I was no guinea pig anatomist, so covering Byron with the drape removed all my landmarks, making it that much harder to choose the spot where I would cut into him.

I made my incision and was soon into the abdomen. The bladder was readily visible because it was extremely inflamed and thickened. Usually a bladder resembles a thin sheet of cling wrap surrounding a pool of water, but this one was almost half a centimetre thick. I had to cut into the bladder to find the stone; however, when my scalpel sliced into it an enormous amount of blood came pouring out – a result of an increased supply to the very angry organ. The blood obscured almost everything. I felt around and was lucky to find the stone on first sweep. We were fairly certain there was only one stone, going by the X-ray, but some stones can be too small to see. So I continued to probe around, knowing that if I left one in we were dooming Byron to more infections down the track.

Meanwhile, Geoff was making hurry-up noises in the corner and when I looked up I realised that he was manually breathing for Byron – lightly squeezing a bag to imitate the normal rate of breathing. Byron had stopped breathing, though his heart was still pumping. This was an extremely dangerous situation and the words of Tom Donnelly were echoing in my head: 'Don't kill the guinea pig with anaesthetic.'

With this in mind, I sewed up the bladder with our finest suture material, checked that it wasn't leaking then stitched up Byron's abdomen and skin. Not long after we switched off the anaesthetic gas, Byron began to move his legs and he was soon up munching on a mouthful of fresh wheaten grass that Myra had provided.

I phoned Myra and again could hear the muffled breathing of Val on the other end of the line too. I informed them of the successful stone removal and Byron's ready recovery from the anaesthetic. They were absolutely ecstatic with the result and I could hear Myra's voice wavering. Val forgot herself and congratulated me over the phone. It was a very rewarding moment.

Two weeks later, when I went to Myra and Val's place to remove the stitches, they were over the moon that he was doing so well – better than they'd seen him in years. I was likewise delighted and relieved. I'd got through by the skin of my teeth, and the less said about it the better.

I was trying to work my way back towards the door, but it was hard given how chatty and happy they were with Byron's improvement.

I didn't want to hang around for any difficult questions like 'How many of these operations had you done in the past?'

'Well, Myra and Val, I'm so glad he's come good. But I really do need to get back to work,' I said.

'Yes, of course. Before you go, though, could you have a quick look at Bessy, the rabbit?'

'Sure.'

'She's got a bloody discharge and she's been a bit lethargic.'

'Has she also been showing signs of aggression?' I asked with growing apprehension.

'Yes, she has actually. It's been really odd. We thought it was because Byron was getting all the attention.'

My heart sank. These were classic symptoms of a uterine tumour. And the treatment was ... surgery.

IF I COULD TALK TO THE ANIMALS

James

After the fiasco of Winston the Pig, Ben and I returned a bit sheepish to the Manilla clinic.

Behind the desk, Suzanne looked concerned: 'Where the hell have you been? I've been trying to cover for you. We've got Mrs Wilson's cat waiting for its blood test and you've got to see a horse out at the Wrights' place on the way home. What happened to you?'

'Nothing,' said Ben, shooting me a glare.

'Nothing,' I agreed.

I think she picked up on the vibe and didn't press the point. Suzanne was a genius at knowing when to interrupt, especially with clients. She knew just when to prompt me, or when to get the dog out the back, away from the client so I had a chance to regroup and think. She was also the best pattern recogniser I've ever come across. She'd hear all the things the client was saying to me and what I was asking the client. Then when I'd pop out the back to get something, she'd appear with a file in her hand. 'Sounds like what we had with Jake Smith's dog a couple of years ago. Here's the file.'

I'd flick through the file, perhaps a little dubious at first, but then I'd see that the symptoms matched exactly. *Hmm, wonder what Tim did here?* So I'd do what Tim had done and it would all come out hunky dory.

Suzanne spent a lot of time in the clinic on her own while I was out on farm visits. Someone would come in: 'My dog's twitching and vomiting and can hardly stand up.'

'Where do you live? ... Oh yeah, you're right on the river.' Her brain would flick through her mental file of similar cases. 'It's probably been bitten by a snake. Let's get some urine and check it out.'

She'd call me and if I couldn't get there she'd tell the client to go to Tamworth or that she could put the dog on a drip herself if they weren't willing to go. I'd get another call saying it was on the drip. Then another saying not to rush back because it was looking heaps better. Suzanne covered for me all the time and made me look good. And she had a great work ethic.

Tamworth was a long way away, so the poor folk of Manilla either got me or they got no one. That helped. Plus the clients had seen many versions of me come and go over the years because Ben always had new grads cycling through.

Over the next two years I worked almost exclusively as the lone vet in Manilla, and the fear gradually subsided. With the help of Suzanne, things almost never went wrong.

Your first job as a new grad can be very stressful. It's all eyes upon you. A hell of a lot of pressure. And the amount of support you get varies. Anthony and I now have the same problem, employing three new grads. They've all got different skills and personalities. You run a fine line between holding their hand too much and stifling them, or not holding it enough. Sometimes they think they don't need help and they do. Sometimes they think they need help and they don't. It's a really difficult line we constantly tread and our first bosses had to tread that line too.

I remember one day early on a guy with a thick Spanish accent came in. His name was 'Sandy' Sanchez, and he was the only Spanish speaker in town. He mumbled something incomprehensible before starting a game of charades. Firstly pointing to himself, 'Me Sandy,' then pointing to the dog, 'Is Pedro,' and finishing with, 'Is seeeeek – not good.' I had to call Jessica in to translate. It wasn't that she understood Spanish, it was just that she was Sandy's neighbour and could understand his English a little better than Suzanne and I.

His strange-looking black-and-white cocker-spaniel/shih tzu cross was clearly sick. Typically a bright and bubbly dog with a massively overshot jaw, which gave him a permanently quizzical expression, Pedro was barely able to raise his head. I looked at him and saw that he had pale gums, and I felt a large irregular mass in his belly – not good. There was a little fluid in the abdomen so I put a needle in and extracted blood – not good either.

I broke the news to Sandy that Pedro had a growth inside his abdomen that was bleeding.

'Is cancer?' Sandy didn't need charades for that one.

'Probably,' I replied, before attaching all the caveats that scientists like to apply – we couldn't be sure unless we performed biopsies, looked for evidence that it might have spread. In essence, though, it was walking like a duck and quacking like a duck so it wasn't likely to be a budgie. I used a lot of words, but I'm pretty sure Sandy only understood one, and that was 'cancer'.

I gave Sandy his options. We could do further investigations and try to understand the lump better with biopsies, ultrasounds and X-rays.

'Not much money,' Sandy replied.

I pantomimed my way through explaining that the most pragmatic option was to anaesthetise Pedro and open his abdomen to see if the mass was a tumour and if it was operable. If it was, great. If not, we'd have to put him to sleep on the table. This was relatively cheap and the only proactive option, given Sandy's budget. Alternatively, we could try to ease his suffering with palliative care, but realistically this meant putting him to sleep now. It was all too much for Sandy, who burst into tears. A whole range of emotions and Spanish words came flying out, none of which made any sense to me except, 'We try, we try.'

We agreed that I would perform the exploratory procedure for a small amount of money. But the odds were not good.

I figured that I'd stabilise Pedro then take him to Barraba so Ben could oversee the surgery. But when I called Ben, he said he was 180 kilometres away. 'I'm away for the next three days bull testing so, um, you're going to have to do it yourself.' He gave me some pointers and encouragement. 'You'll be right. You can spay a dog. And if you can do that, anything else is either going to be simple or it's not going to be operable. See what you find.'

So I opened Pedro up for an exploratory laparotomy, which is a fancy way of saying I was having a look around in the abdomen. Regardless, I felt like I was totally winging it. The dog was on its back and I made the cut down its middle. The hole I made was big, from near the spot where the ribs join to where the pubic bone starts.

'Shit! Are you planning on getting your whole head in there?' Suzanne joked, breaking some of the tension. I needed this hole to be big so I could have a really good look around and understand what was going on. It didn't take long. Ideally, you're looking for healthy pink tissue, but I was seeing ugly dark-red to almost-black lumps spread through the liver and the spleen. The intestines, which should be quite mobile, were stuck to the cancerous masses. Deep in the abdomen, towards the spine, there is a fixed point called 'the root of mesentery' where some organs, blood vessels and lymph nodes reside. It was just horrendous there. That was the mass that I'd been able to feel from the outside; now I was face to face with it – and it was ugly. There were irregular black lobules bursting out of the wrapping of the lymph nodes and organs, like what you see on the cigarette packets.

I'd seen these sorts of operations through my final year so it wasn't especially shocking for me. But it was going to be hard to tell Sandy that poor old Pedro had cancer everywhere. Even if Sandy was the richest man in the world and I was the best surgeon, we could not have bought Pedro more than a few weeks' grace.

I called Sandy to break the news. It was my first such call. I knew that it was important to be clear and concise. I had Suzanne bring over the phone and put it on speaker. 'Sandy, Pedro is in surgery and I'm very sorry to tell you, it's bad news. There is a lot of invasive cancer and there's nothing we can do to save him ... he's simply riddled with it.'

In these situations, you have to make sure the client understands the gravity of the situation but at the same time show empathy. I suspect, however, that after the initial bad news Sandy didn't take much else in.

He had braced himself for the worst. Through his sobs we heard him say: 'Put him to sleep.'

Once you've made that phone call you no longer have to worry about being sterile. I drew up the injection and put Pedro to sleep, knowing that it was the best thing for him and that I'd done all I could. After that I had to stitch him up and make him presentable so poor old Sandy could take him home to bury. He could barely speak when he came in. He hugged me for a long time.

We did a lot of emergency work at Manilla. It seemed to have an inordinate number of dogs hit by cars, chest traumas, pyothorax – pus in the chest cavity – and lots of snakebites. One day a couple of battlers, Paddy and Lynne Whiteley, came in with their little Jack Russell, Chuckie. Chuckie was weak, unable to stand, panting and convulsing. It wasn't hard to diagnose with all the dual punctures on his neck. Jack Russells are the poster dogs of snake killers but if you take that up as a profession it's just a matter of time before you become the poster dog of snakebite victims. This was the second time Chuckie had found himself on the wrong end of the fangs. My predecessor, Tim, had treated him a year or two earlier, but judging by the files this time seemed far worse.

The first thing was to give him some sedation to calm him down and then get an IV line in. Not a difficult task and one of the basics of veterinary medicine, but a challenge when the dog is convulsing and the pressure is on. Once that catheter was in, though, I was in control, and the sedation started to kick in. I administered drugs to reduce the reaction to the bite and guard against reactions to the anti-venom – cortisone, anti-histamines, adrenalin and antibiotics. He was very close to death when I gave him the anti-venom and got the mask over his snout to give him oxygen.

After that initial treatment, we wrapped a cage in Glad Wrap and put him in there, pumping it full of oxygen to maintain the 'oxygen therapy'. He was terribly sick and we worked long and hard to save him, nursing him through the night, but by morning he was much better. That's the thing about brown-snake venom: it is exceedingly lethal, but if it doesn't kill the animal, they bounce back very quickly. By the time Paddy and Lynne came in the next morning to check on him, Chuckie was up and jumping around like a new dog. I tried to tell them that what I had done was all standard procedure – oxygen, anti-venom and fluids – nothing groundbreaking. It was just a matter of being attentive. Nevertheless, they thought the sun shone out of my large intestine.

The day before, while we'd hovered over Chuckie's limp little body, we'd chatted for a long while, and I'd got to know and like the couple. They were both in their early fifties, both grey-haired and a little frumpy, with a classic larrikin streak about them. They'd told me about their pet cockatoo named Cocky, who Lynne had inherited from her father some thirty years earlier. Cockatoos can live to be 100, so you don't just have them for life; you have them for your children's and grandchildren's lives as well.

'It's got a big lump on its leg,' Lynne had said. 'We've never brought it into the vet before because I don't reckon there's anything you blokes could do about it anyway.'

'Yeah, birds aren't my forte,' I'd said. 'But maybe you could see a specialist about it.'

They'd let the conversation slide, but now with Chuckie running around like it was open-day at the butcher they brought the subject of the cockatoo up again.

'You seem to be pretty good at this vetting caper,' Paddy said. 'I reckon you could probably fix Cocky's leg too.'

Bird medicine and surgery was the last exam we ever sat at uni (with the black-tie theme), and I chose to take a glass-half-full view of my results in that subject. I scored 51 per cent – representing an impeccable balance between no desire to study and the need to pass. Rumour has it that our bird lecturer didn't even read the exam papers; he just gave you the mark he thought you deserved. I took from my 51 that he probably didn't like me but was happy to see the back of me. Luckily it didn't cost me getting honours, but we did graduate in academic order and the person who graduated one spot in front of me reminds me about it just about every day at work. I didn't tell Paddy and Lynne any of that; just quietly wished I had been more studious in those avian subjects.

'I'm happy to have a look,' I said, 'but there is a bird specialist in Tamworth. He only sees birds. He'll know a lot more about this. You should see him.'

'No, no. We want you to see Cocky,' said Lynne.

'Okay, bring him in. I can have a look.' So they brought Cocky in on the back of their ute. He needed such heavy-duty transport because his cage was huge, probably 2 metres wide by 2 metres tall. Fortunately, the clinic was a small hut built inside a huge shed so they were able to drive into the shed, right up to the clinic and squeeze him into the only room that fitted his cage, the waiting room.

'Can you get him out?' I asked.

Cocky might have lived with them for thirty years but I could see they hadn't handled him much. Eventually they threw a towel over him and I had to stick my hand into the towel to try to pull him out. As he wriggled and flapped in there, he proved to be most effective at piercing my glove with his powerful jaws. One of the interesting things about cockatoos and galahs is that their tracheal rings (the solid bits of their windpipe) are completely made of bone. While humans have soft cartilage in the windpipe making them easy to choke, Cocky and his brethren have complete circular rings of bone that make it impossible to choke them. So I took advantage of this and squeezed his neck hard to stop the little beggar making mincemeat of my hand, in the full knowledge his eyes weren't going to pop out of his skull.

Suzanne grabbed his wings and secured them in a towel, allowing me to inspect the leg where I saw a significant lump. I was blatantly honest. 'Look, he's got a tumorous growth. I don't know what it is. I don't know much about it. I could probably take it off but the anaesthetic would be very tricky and you'd be better off seeing the bird guy in Tamworth. I reckon he could get it off blindfolded.'

'You could take it off,' Paddy said.

'I don't have the right anaesthetic equipment.'

'But you said before that you could do it,' Lynne said.

'Well, I've got gear that would do the job, but it's far riskier than if I had the specialised bird equipment. That's why you're better off with this guy in Tamworth. He'd sort it out in no time. It's half an hour's drive. We could put Cocky in a smaller cage.'

They weren't buying it. They really thought that since I saved their dog I was the man for the job. They had suspicious eyes, Paddy and Lynne, but I had obviously passed their scrutiny.

How am I going to get out of this?

'How much would it cost for the guy in Tamworth to do it?'

'Oh, it'd probably be less than $100.' I tried to make it sound very attractive.

'How much for you to do it?'

'Because I don't have the gear, it's going to take significantly longer. It'll also be riskier. It's gunna be probably $350 for me to do it. It's cheaper to go to Tamworth to see the guy who's got the gear and the knowledge. Here, let me put Cocky in a cage for you.'

Paddy and Lynne exchanged glances. 'Nah, we want you to do it.'

I realised I was stuck. I'd given them a quote and they'd accepted. *Damn.*

'Okay then, I guess … umm … leave him … with me and I'll … sort him out.'

'Great, thanks mate. Can we come back and get him about 4.30?'

So Suzanne popped Cocky back into his massive penthouse apartment in the waiting room where he happily talked to the rest of the clients. 'Hello, whadayawant? Hello, whadayawant?'

I got through the morning consults and it came time to anaesthetise the bird. Suzanne and I caught him a bit more efficiently this time and wrapped him in vet wrap, a type of bandage that doesn't stick to skin or feathers – just to itself – like Glad Wrap for animals. I put a mask on him and he quickly went to sleep. The main difference between me and the specialist, aside from his greater skill and knowledge, was that he had specialised bird anaesthetic gas that was safer for them. So we kept our anaesthetic light. We didn't want it to kill him.

The tumour was large, down on the lower part of the leg which is just skin and bone. But it bulged out in such a way that the normal skin was quite close together on either side. I was able to get in under the tumour with scissors, cut it away, then stitch the skin back together without much fuss. It all fell into place rather nicely. I put absorbable stitches in so we wouldn't have to knock him out again to take them out. I was pretty chuffed with myself. We turned the anaesthetic off, unwrapped Cocky in a dark quiet room and waited for him to gradually wake.

As he came to, Cocky's eyes started to flicker. His sulphur crest flared. He looked at Suzanne and looked at me. 'Alo,' he croaked; a deep throaty croak. We cracked up. Our patients don't normally talk to us. It seemed so wonderfully ridiculous. 'Helloooo,' he said, clearer now. Coming to life for his audience. 'What's going on here? What's going on here?'

With huge smiles on our faces, feeling like Dr Doolittles, we put him back in the waiting room. I went to write up the bill and faced a dilemma. *How the hell can I charge them $350 for this?* It had all been so straightforward. The quote I'd made up was just to deter them from having me do the surgery. I felt really guilty because I liked them. So, with a warm inner glow, I wrote $150.

But the feeling was not entirely reciprocated. When a little old lady, Mrs Eileen James, came in with her dachshund, Schnitzel, I came out to see them in the waiting room.

'Fucking arsehole,' someone yelled.

At first I thought it was Mrs James. I was taken aback. Then I realised it wasn't a person at all.

'Fucking arsehole,' Cocky said again, clear as day.

'Just ignore good ol' Cocky here,' I said to Mrs James. 'He's a bit upset over an earlier medical procedure. Please, follow me to the consult room.'

'Fucking arsehole. Fucking arsehole,' Cocky called out as I led her as quickly as possible away.

For the rest of the afternoon, as soon as I walked out to greet new patients, Cocky would see me and let fly with a cacophony of blue language. It was not really the look we were going for. I had to ring Lynne. 'The operation was a success. But can you please come and get Cocky now. He's doing terrible things to our business.'

There was definitely a downside to being Dr Doolittle.

A VERY EXPENSIVE 24-CARAT GOLDFISH

Anthony

Not long after my experience with Byron the guinea pig, the clinic received a message asking for someone to make a house call on a fish. Unsurprisingly, the job was passed down the line to me. I've got to admit, even I thought this was a little off beat. I gave the clients a call. 'Can you bring the fish into the clinic in its tank?' I asked.

'No, no. He's in a pond,' said an elderly man's voice down the line.

'Right. So he's outdoors?'

'Yes. And we don't want to catch him because we think it will distress him. He's never been in a tank in his life.'

'Okay, I'll come and see you,' I said, trying to mask my reluctance. I mean, people who have goldfish in their ponds don't tend to do much for them other than scoop them out when they go belly up. But I'd learnt a lot from Byron the guinea pig. If people wanted veterinary care for their pets it was my duty to give it, and give it to the best of my ability. And it was immensely rewarding to work with people who cared so deeply about their animals.

I pulled up at the house with a positive attitude. The elderly couple were waiting for me on the porch of their 1980s brick dwelling. By the time I'd turned into the driveway and pulled the handbrake on, they were at the side of the Magna ready to take me to the patient. I grabbed my bag like I was a professional fish guy and refrained from making any jokes about having hooks and sinkers in there.

They introduced themselves as Alice and Bill.

'What's wrong with the fish?' I asked.

'If we knew what was wrong with the fish we wouldn't be calling you,' Bill said.

I hate that answer, but you wear it because you know people get prickly when they are worried.

'Is it a pet?'

'No, no. We just noticed there was something wrong with it.'

They led me around the back where the pond was situated under a pretty pergola. I saw there were quite a few goldfish in there, all nicely protected from cats and birds by faded green fly-wire strung over thick steel reo. The water was dirty so you couldn't see anything down deep, but all the fish cooperated by coming to the surface.

Anybody who uses the phrase 'the memory of a goldfish' has never had a goldfish. Everybody who has had a goldfish knows that when you approach the tank all the goldfish immediately come to the surface to be fed. So they must have the ability to remember events. If goldfish had the thirty-second memory that popular myth says they have, they would have forgotten the fact that your appearing at the tank signals the arrival of food.

When the fish realised no food was coming, they got bored and returned to the depths, leaving just one on the surface. He was big for a goldfish, about 10 centimetres long, floating on his side, right side up. When I approached, he dived down with all the others, but then he couldn't seem to stay there and soon floated back to the surface, with the right side again coming to the top. I could see he had a distended growth there.

'He is our oldest fish,' Bill said. 'We got him when we first moved in twenty-six years ago. We hope he is not in any pain.'

'I don't know what the growth is, but given his age it could be a tumour,' I said. 'In order to find out for sure, I'd have to catch him and take him back to the practice to have a better look. I'm not sure what it is, but it's obviously affecting his buoyancy.'

Alice and Bill were probably in their late seventies. They were both short. Bill wore beaten-up brown leather shoes under trousers belonging to a suit that would have been new two generations ago. Alice was in a floral dress with a cardigan. She wore a concerned look on her face.

'We're worried he's in pain or distress,' she said.

'I don't think you need to be worried about that. He's still eating happily. He's still interacting with the other fish and able to submerge himself if he has to. He's not floating on the surface like a balloon. And even if he was he's protected by the mesh.'

At uni, we spent less than a minute every day studying fish, and that was at the canteen when you were deciding whether to go the fish sticks or the chicken. We did actually do some fish lectures but the topic wasn't prioritised. It was done as a stream when we were living at Camden, which was a pretty wild time so we didn't always attend. The fish lecturers were people who came in from outside so you never had the chance to bond with them or the subject either.

But don't let it ever be said that we don't have empathy for fish at the Berry vet clinic. When we did our 'Blinding Nemo' end-of-fourth-year revue, someone made a Nemo suit which James wore to the fish markets at Pyrmont. He walked through the car park yelling, 'Eating fish is murder.' On the way back we went to McDonald's and in the Drive Thru he was in the back of the ute, wearing this clownfish costume, trying to converse with the poor teenager serving us: 'I can't believe you serve fillet of fish here. Can you understand how that makes me feel, as a fish? I mean, put yourself in my flippers …'

One of the things I did remember from uni was how to anaesthetise a fish, because I thought that was really cool. You get the fish in a smallish tank and you put the anaesthetic in the water and the fish passes out from it. But how do you do surgery with the fish asleep in a tank? You can't. You put the fish on a big sponge and place a tube in the fish's mouth, pumping the anaesthetised water in so it flows out through its gills into the sponge. The water flows down into a receptacle and back to the tank. Then, when you want to wake the fish up you take the pump out of the anaesthetised tank and put it into a fresh-water one and pump that through instead. As the fish starts to wake you slip it into the fresh-water tank.

I thought that was awesome. So I was keen to give it a try – if the fish did have a tumour and if Alice and Bill wanted to try to save it. I gave them their options. Euthanasia, surgery or letting nature take its course. After tossing up the options they decided they'd keep an eye on it for now and wait until it got so bad it could no longer submerge itself at all. We'd decide what to do then.

I walked out thinking, 'How can I charge for that?' It was just a chat, but we have to charge for our time and knowledge. So I sent them a small bill because that's what Geoff and Geoff were paying me for. I didn't expect to hear from Alice and Bill again. I thought that when the time came, they'd just scoop it out with a net and leave it in the air to die. But we got a call about two months later and they asked to see me specifically – which tended to get up the Geoffs' noses a bit. 'Why are people asking to see the junior?' they'd ask. Then they'd hear it was about a fish and they'd laugh and be glad I was the name on those people's speed dials.

'We think it's time to put the fish to sleep,' Bill said. 'He can't submerge at all any more. He's constantly on the surface.'

'Okay,' I said. 'It's fairly simple. You can just scoop him out and hit him on the head, or you can move him into a separate tank medicated with clove oil. The clove oil is a natural anaesthetic and he'll peacefully go to sleep and not wake up.'

'No, we don't want to do that. We want you to come out and put him down but not that way. We want you to give him an injection because we don't like the idea of him suffering.'

I turned up with a net and a 5-litre bucket with a lid. Only Bill was there to greet me this time and he led me back around to the pond. I caught the fish and took some of its pond water. The lump on the side of the fish had almost doubled in size since my last visit. On the way out the gate Bill told me that Alice had taken a turn for the worse and they were being forced to move to a facility where she could be cared for. He wanted to stay near her so they were selling the family home and moving to a retirement home. As I left I could see the redness in Bill's eyes and the odd stray tear; the fish was one last connection to a more hopeful time, twenty-six years earlier.

I took the fish back to work, running the gauntlet of raised eyebrows and rolling eyes as I came back through with my heavy bucket. I scooped it out of the bucket and injected Lethabarb into its abdomen, placing it back into the bucket and watching it slow down till the life was gone. It was the most expensive goldfish in Berry after two house calls, a euthanasia and a burial, but it was also the best example of how compassionate people can be; that they would spend the time and the money to do this for an animal they said they had no bond with. It didn't even have a name.

Alice and Bill had tied up a loose end and I never heard from them again.

RODEO CLOWNS

James

The grey gelding came down the race with its head erect and nostrils flaring. Its pupils were dilated and its eyes flashed anger, like the guy in the corner of the pub itching for a fight at 1 a.m. His name was Destroyer and this is what he was bred for: to buck humans into the middle of next week. Horses like this are worth a lot of money and are looked after accordingly.

Fortunately, the new grad, Mark, and I weren't there to ride him for eight seconds (there was no risk of that happening). We just wanted to stitch up the gash in his flank and leave quietly with no hoof prints in our skulls.

I had survived my first year at Barraba, growing in skill and confidence, and now Mark was here to experience what I'd been through the year before. But instead of calling Ben when he had a problem, he usually called me because I was a little less intimidating and talked in full sentences. So I'd dragged him along to this prime rodeo stud in the Horton Valley knowing that I'd probably need a hand, or at least someone to hold mine, as I dealt with these fearsome beasts.

We did a lot of work in the Horton Valley to the west of Barraba. It was prime agricultural land, and if you approached it from Barraba via the Trevallyn Road you dropped into a magnificent vista of rich, green fertile land – some of the most valuable in Australia. The valley was populated by big characters and by little ponies belonging to the children of some of the richest people in the country. There was also a strong rodeo community that centred around the little township of Upper Horton, which held a famous New Year's Eve rodeo.

The people who owned the bucking Destroyer had him in the race, which was an effective restraint for now. But the thing about that was it signalled to him he was about to be ridden and that it was time to deal with these pesky humans. It was game on.

Working with rodeo people fills you with a sense of ineptitude in the bravery department. There is an element of the Wild West in how they talk, walk and act, and as much as I'd never pretend to do what they do, I still didn't want to seem scared in front of them.

With Destroyer restrained, I managed to jam an 18-gauge needle into his rump muscle in more of a stabbing motion than with the controlled precision I'd normally demand, but the sedative got in. Once his ears started to droop and the fire started to leave his eyes, I was able to carefully and quickly get the anaesthetic into the jugular vein without getting my fingers crushed. They were huge doses because Destroyer was so keyed up. This was a pampered, valuable horse, but he didn't return the love. Destroyer was pampered and valued precisely because he wasn't friendly to humans – those that tried to ride him and, as it turned out, those who tried to stick needles into him.

Once the anaesthetic was in we let him out of the chute, just in time for him to fall to the ground and go to sleep. Usually that process is carefully stage-managed, the vet controlling the head rope to ensure as gentle a passage as possible to the ground, but with rodeo stock you stand well clear and let them sort it out for themselves. Destroyer teetered and went down, allowing us to get to work. It was all very routine in the end. We cleaned the unruly gash and pulled it together into a neat wound. And we made sure we used dissolvable sutures so we wouldn't be called back to remove them.

Before we'd finished stitching him up, we got a call to go to a nearby property for a problem calving. So we changed out of our overalls and waited for Destroyer to wake up then headed off to the calving. It turned out to be caesarean so I let Mark do that one, and it went without a hitch.

Once again, before we'd had a chance to clean ourselves up my phone rang. This time it was a bloated bull, which again had defied Murphy's Law by being located just a few kilometres down the road. So we changed out of our overalls and drove over.

The farmer, Jason McKay, came out to greet us. He was relatively young for a farmer, probably in his early thirties, with big red hands and a checked shirt that matched his blue eyes. 'Yeah, my bull's looking like he's ready to burst,' Jason explained, taking off his Akubra to wipe his brow and revealing a bone-white forehead atop his otherwise red-brown face.

He led us towards the yards. 'I only got him a few months ago. He's worth a packet. I was just riding past him this morning when I noticed he wasn't right.'

I didn't have to look very hard to see that this was quite possibly the largest bull I'd ever laid eyes on. It was a South Devon. South Devons are already the largest of all the British breeds of cattle, but this deep-red bull was a big one of his type, and on top of that he was so impossibly bloated you couldn't help thinking a pinprick might send him whirling through the sky like an unleashed party balloon.

Ruminants like cows and sheep have big fermenting vats as their first stomachs. If they eat too much clover or lucerne when they're not used to it, it can send the whole process awry, bloating them until there's so much pressure on their lungs they die from suffocation. I thought that might be the case here.

'What type of pasture's he been on?' I asked.

'Just ordinary old grass,' Jason said. 'Nothing different at all.'

Bloat happens for a few reasons. When it's caused by what they've eaten, the gas is suspended in a froth throughout the rumen, making it difficult to release with a stomach tube, so you have to perform a rumenotomy. If something else has caused the bloat, like an obstruction, the gas sits on top of the rumen and so can be relieved with the tube. We needed to have a good look.

Mark and I changed back into our overalls. We set to work getting the bull into a position where we could examine him. This fellow would have struggled to fit up the race on a normal day. There was no way we could get him up there as he was now. So we coaxed him towards the race and got his head into the narrow passage, then shut a gate behind him leaving him somewhat restrained. Whether it was his exploding guts or his natural temperament, he remained placid.

We clambered over the rails and I hung over the gate to get to, his tail in relative safety to inject a sedative. Sedating cattle is always a double-edged sword because some are very sensitive to the sedative xylazine and can fall over. You're always cautious about how much to give, but we needed this monster to be well restrained for what we were about to do to him.

Jason got a head collar on him, something he was probably used to, as he had been a show bull. He wasn't overly distressed. We examined him closely and listened – there was almost no ruminal noise and when I pinged my finger against his belly I could hear a noise like a bouncing basketball. Sometimes you can hear this noise with a stethoscope and we use it to diagnose gas in certain areas in the abdomen. In this case Mark heard it from a few metres away – no stethoscope required.

The bull was still breathing okay and still calm. We thought it reasonable to try to pass a stomach tube in to see if we could release some gas. If it worked it would also be a simple way to get some anti-bloat oil into him and that might be the end of the story. With his head tied in the halter I was able to get a set of nose pliers – blunt instruments that pincer together in the nostrils – on him giving additional restraint of the head. I was standing in the race in front of the bull, a scary spot to be, but given how bloated he was I knew it was safer than it felt. There was no way he could squeeze through to where I was.

I put about half a metre of black irrigation pipe, commonly called polypipe, into his mouth and over his tongue to stop him biting the tube I was about to insert. Then I threaded the delicate tube through the pipe.

'Geez, that's a fairly serious weapon,' mumbled Jason, clearly not a fan of observing medical procedures.

The tube passed easily down the bull's throat and into his rumen but there was little of the hoped-for 'whoosh' of gas. Instead a strange coloured fluid dribbled out. I inspected it as it hit the dirt and noticed a little black ball about the size of a pea wedged into the end of the tube. *Interesting.* I got the ball out and had a closer look. It appeared to be plant matter but beyond that I couldn't tell what it was. I had a closer look at the fluid in the dirt and saw three more little balls lying there.

'This might be what he's eaten,' I said, showing them to Jason. 'Do you know what it is?'

'I got no idea. Never seen it before.'

The bull, meanwhile, was continuing to inflate. Normally bloat makes the left side of the animal bulge outwards, but when it gets really bad the bulge comes out the right side too. And this one was definitely starting to come out both sides. On top of that, we were seeing signs of distress in his breathing.

'We'd better do a rumenotomy. What do you think, Mark?'

'I think so.' There was a hint of resignation in his voice; it was just on dusk and the end of a big day for both of us. Unfortunately there was no option but to suck it up and get on with the job.

A rumenotomy is basically a stab into the rumen to relieve the pressure. We use a trocar, which is essentially a metal tube with a pointy end and a handle. We had a little bit of time as this bull was still fairly stable, but we were out of light. Jason fetched us a torch and I asked him to shine it on the site as we shaved the skin and gave it a quick scrub, before instilling a bit of local. I made an incision to start with for a bit of a peek and shriek. Mark grasped the tissues and held them out so that nothing could spill into the abdominal cavity. Again, there was nothing in the way of a pleasing 'whoosh' of gas, but some fluid containing more of those mysterious black balls ran out. *This is weird. What are these things?* It was hard to see them because the torchlight was nowhere near where we were working.

A quick glance back towards Jason revealed a man who was clearly queasy at the sight of blood. He looked as pale as smoke.

'You all right, mate?' I asked.

'Fine,' he managed through gritted teeth. 'I just can't look at that shit. It's messed up.'

'Okay, just try and keep the light on this area. Lean it on the post and keep your weight on it, then you won't have to look.' I think that gave him something to focus on – not moving and certainly not looking.

I decided we'd better make a bigger hole to get a better look. This animal weighed more than a tonne – about the same as a Toyota Corolla. On a normal day, his rumen would have been about the size of a 44-gallon drum, but it was much bigger today with all the bloat. So carving into his side was no small matter. I cut my way in through the leathery hide, splitting the muscles with scissors and working my way down into the rumen. The harsh smell of putrefaction from that huge fermenting vat overcame the pleasant background aroma of grass clippings.

I was losing my light again. 'Hey Jason. A bit to the left,' I called out. 'Yep. Up a bit and back to the right. That's good.'

I still couldn't see much so I dipped my hand in and scooped out a palmful of the fluid. My hand was covered with those pea-sized black balls. *Crikey! What am I dealing with?*

Mark continued to hold the rumen while I tacked it to the skin, allowing us easy access and freeing Mark up to take the torch from Jason because I knew he wasn't up for what I had in mind. As Mark shone the light inside the rumen I saw that the balls weren't just sitting on the top of the fluid; they were evenly suspended all the way through. The only explanation I could come up with was that, whatever they were, they had created a large 'osmotic gradient'; sucking all this fluid out of the blood and tissues and into the stomach.

We didn't know what they were but we were now pretty sure we'd found the cause of the problem. I just had to get them out of the rumen and we'd be right. I started scooping them by hand but I soon realised there was no way this would get them all out. The rumen was so big I couldn't even reach the lower portions of it.

I grabbed some tubing, figuring I could siphon the fluid and balls out. I put one end of the tube into the rumen and was about to put the other end to my mouth when I noticed Jason's painful grimace.

'What are you doing?' he asked.

'We're setting up a siphon to get these balls out.'

'Ahhh, I can't look.' He hid his eyes behind his forearm. This big fat dusty farmer with skin as leathery as his Akubra was like a kid watching a scary movie. I put the tube to my lips and sucked on it, being careful to get it out of my mouth before the gut contents hit me in the throat. It flowed well for a few seconds before the balls blocked it up. We tried again, but the tube kept blocking. This wasn't going to work.

It looked like we had to go back to doing it by hand.

'What are you doing now?' Jason asked.

'Fishing them out with our hands.'

'Oh no. I can't watch.' His red complexion was glowing in the fading light.

Mark and I scooped away, vigorously at first, but there were thousands of the balls and we hardly made a dent. After about half an hour, Mark jacked up. 'This is useless', he said. 'We're never going to get them out.'

'Yeah, you're right,' I said. 'But I don't see that we've got any choice.'

We fell into defeated silence. 'Have you got anything here on the farm that we might be able to use?' I asked Jason.

'I don't know. Can't look. Can't look.'

The flash came to me gently, like a low-watt bulb being switched on.

'Have you got a diesel pump?' I asked.

'Yeah. It's not clean though.'

'Doesn't matter. It's going inside his stomach. It's not clean in there either. Have you seen how freaking dirty this is?'

'No I haven't. And I don't intend to either.'

'Can you just bring the pump over?'

A lot of farms store their diesel in 44-gallon drums. To get to it, they use pumps that have a solid metal pipe dropping to the bottom of the drum. Jason was having a good chuckle to himself as he brought over one such contraption that was powered by a wind-up handle. 'You gunna put that in my bull?'

'You got a better idea?'

Mark went and got a towel from the car. He pegged it to the top of a 20-litre plastic bucket. It was going to act as a filter. We needed to remove the balls but keep the fluid, because the bull was going to want it back. He needed the liquid part, but more so he needed the community of bacteria that lived in it. Ruminants don't live on grass itself. When they swallow grass it feeds the microbes in their rumen and those microbes then produce the nutrients that the cow or bull needs to survive. If we took this bull's bugs and replaced them with plain water, it would almost certainly kill him.

I picked up the pump and dropped the pipe into the bull's rumen, and with both of us holding the pump steady we started to wind the handle. Fluid filled with these balls started gushing out in spurts onto the towel and through into the bucket. I'd stop pumping and Mark would clean the balls away, then we'd resume. After we pumped about half the rumen out, I pulled the pump out of the bull and put it in the bucket. We then proceeded to pump the fluid from the bucket back into the bull, before reversing the process again. We did that three or four times until there were virtually no balls coming through any more. We filled him up one last time. His rumen was about half the size it had been and he looked far less misshapen. His breathing was on the improve and he looked to be brightening up. Mark sewed up his rumen, reinserted it, then sewed up his muscle and skin, and we gave him plenty of antibiotics and anti-inflammatories.

We let the bull out of his makeshift crush and he wandered back into the holding yard behind the race, looking pretty relaxed. Jason threw him some hay to tide him over until morning.

We got back in the car and drove home marvelling at our success and creativity. We rang Jason the next day and he reported the bull was doing just fine. 'But, geez, you guys are pretty wild putting a diesel pump inside a bull.'

'Not wild at all. Just mild-mannered vets doing our job.'

The bull survived his ordeal just fine. I sent a sample of the black balls off to a lab but they were unable to identify them. A few months later I heard that he broke his leg fighting another bull and had to be put down. Such is life on the farm.

ONE OF THE FAMILY

Anthony

I've never considered myself a cat or a dog person; I've always loved both. When I was a kid, my sister and I really wanted a dog. But Mum and Dad worked long hours and didn't feel that it was fair to have one, given all the time dogs demand. Even then I could see it was a sensible decision but it didn't stop us nagging.

I was about ten or eleven years old when we lost our family cat, Wilton. Dad relented to the badgering and went to buy us a dog. He had a black labrador earmarked but he got there and decided it was a bad idea and backed out. I'd begged to go with him but wisely he wouldn't take me. There was no way I would have let him leave that place without a dog on our leash.

Soon after, we were driving to the farm from Sydney and just before we got there, Dad saw a sign at the Old Toolijooa Schoolhouse advertising kittens for sale. He didn't say anything about it to us, though, and when the opportunity arose he ducked out of the house to have a look at them.

At this stage in life, I was glued to Dad's side. Whatever farm work was being done, or whatever else he was doing, I had to be there helping.

So when I realised he'd jumped in the car and driven off without me, I was filthy.

I stormed up to Mum. 'Where's Dad?'

'He's just ducked into town.'

'Why's he ducked into town? Why wasn't I allowed to go?'

'He's just gone to the co-op,' she said.

'I want to go to the co-op. I love going to the co-op. I wanted to go to the co-op.'

I was absolutely beside myself, displaying all the nagging skills that Dad was so wise to escape on the dog trip, and I continued on in my rage until I heard the car return. I shot out to the garage to give him a piece of my mind. 'Where have you been? Why wasn't I allowed to come?'

'Look, I've got something to show you,' he said.

We went to the back of the Range Rover and he opened it to reveal a cat carrier holding two blue-point Siamese kittens. My anger evaporated. 'Oh Dad! Where did you get them?'

Before he could answer, I heard Mum's voice from the other end of the house: 'Them? What do you mean "them"?'

'Honey, I couldn't choose between them. The big one was so relaxed and floppy and sooky, but the little one was so in-your-face and purring and wanting attention, I couldn't decide. Stuff it, I thought, I'll get both.'

We were in the car back home to Sydney at the end of the weekend with the kittens in the cat carrier on the back seat. Mum turned to my sister, Jackie, and me. 'You guys had better come up with names for these kittens. One can be Anthony's and one can be Jackie's.' We thought about it for a while and I plucked the name Wesley Thomas Bennett from somewhere, and Jackie, who must have been about seven, named hers Stuart Charles Bennett.

Mum was like, 'Okay ... They're very formal. What about something like Snookems or Diddems or Silky?'

'No. I like Wesley,' I said.

'And I like Stuart,' said Jackie. And that was it. The names stuck and they never let us name a pet again.

Siamese cats demand attention, so Stuart and Wesley were like dogs. They'd follow us everywhere. They'd come to the farm with us, and when Dad and I were out moving cows, you'd turn around and see their two tails poking through the long grass as they followed us – even when we were kilometres from the house. You'd be right up the back of the property with no idea the cats had seen us leave, and then you'd hear a noise – something like the distant whine of a chainsaw. That was their version of a meow.

We'd pretend they'd herd the cows like sheepdogs though they were much more hindrance than help. The cows found them so fascinating that they'd stop going where they were meant to go and come back for a sniff and a look. If we could have got the cats in front of the herd they would have been much more useful; the cows would have happily followed them anywhere.

So these cats were a big part of our lives. Wesley was the big sooky one with a very laid-back personality. Stuart had a lot more aggression and ticker. Stuart was the boss, except when food was around. Stuart could bash Wesley up all day, have him cowering on the dining room chair, too afraid to move, but bring dinner out and Wesley was like the Incredible Hulk. He'd just change into a scary monster cat.

One day towards the end of high school, I got home from school during a heavy rain storm. I saw Wesley outside under the clothesline in the tiled courtyard taking a pelting from the heavy, soaking raindrops.

Gee, that's weird for him to be out in this and not moving.

The rain was so heavy he was lying in an inch of water on the tiles. His fur was spiked out from the wet. As I approached, I saw blood and gouges on his torso, and I knew he'd been mauled by something. His body was cold and rigid when I picked him up. With a sense of horror and helplessness that was new to me, I took him inside and phoned Dad at work. Dad would know what to do.

'There's nothing you can do,' Dad said. 'If he's dead, he's dead. Maybe you could think about burying him, or if that's too difficult you can leave him and I'll bury him when I get home.' I thought about it and decided it was something I wanted to do. It was very sad but I guess it was part of that healing process. I dug a hole and laid him in it, holding a sodden little ceremony in my head, then just sat out in the rain for a while, thinking about Wesley and the way he left us. I had a bit of a cry. I was fragile for months.

I got home from school the next day. We had a steep driveway that went down towards the river and bush all around us. There were cement stairs through the bush, to the neighbour's house higher up the slope. I remember coming down the driveway and looking back up to my left into the bush and there was the prime suspect, the neighbour's brown kelpie cross. Coming back for seconds. Blood boiled in me. I saw a quarter brick and reached for it. I was pretty sporty and had a good arm. I went to throw the brick and the dog took off up the stairs when he saw my arm go back. At the last minute I changed my mind. I realised I couldn't hammer a dog with a brick. I didn't want to hurt it. As upset as I was, I knew it wasn't the dog's fault. It was in the dog's nature to chase cats. I threw to miss and yelled, the brick cracking into the step behind it.

The dog never came back. And Stuart Charles Bennett became an indoor cat after that. We never let him out. I suppose Wesley's loss made Stuart an even more valued member of the family. He was always on us and with us. I remember driving to the snow when I was in second year at uni. James was there, along with our other good friends Alex, Mitch and Kate. The circle of friends was consolidating into a tight group by then, but we were still getting to know each other.

I was chatting away about Stuart and I said, 'He's such a fussy eater he'll only eat Hill's pet food.'

'What are you talking about?' Kate said, somewhat incredulous. 'Stuart eats cat food?'

'Yeah. Why wouldn't he?'

'How do your parents allow it?'

'They're the ones that give it to him.'

And then she twigged that she was missing something. 'Stuart is your brother, isn't he?'

'He's our cat.'

'But you talk about him like he's your brother, like he's a family member.'

'Well, he is a family member. Stuart Charles Bennett.'

WHO YOU GUNNA CALL?

James

The phone rang at 5 a.m. 'James. James. Wake up. Get out of bed.' The voice was urgent, rapid, faking pain.

'I'm up,' I said.

'You're a liar. As if you'd be up this early on a Sunday.' It was Wayne McAndrew, a local dairy farmer that everyone called Mook. I knew him well from touch footy and cricket and it seemed that he knew me even better. I have a reflex where if someone calls me at 3 a.m. and says, 'Sorry for waking you.' I say, 'No, no, I'm awake.' It comes from me never having liked getting out of bed as a kid and Mum devoting hours to getting me up to go to school. She'd be at the door yelling at me and I'd just reflexively lie, 'No, no, I'm awake,' and promptly go back to sleep. The words would come from my mouth before I even realised.

Wayne had got me out of bed before so he knew the procedure: startle me. 'Get out of bed, you lazy bastard. I've got a prolapsed cow.'

We had a final-year student, Jandy, staying with us. She was doing the weekend on call with me, so I sleepily shuffled down the hall and knocked on her door. 'Jandy, get up. We've got to go see a cow.'

We drove to Mook's place in that early Sunday morning fug, but Mook, like so many dairy farmers, seemed to have inexhaustible energy. 'Come on, I've been up for hours.'

The cow had calved in the middle of a blackberry bush and then the uterus had followed the calf out. A prolapse. The uterus was hanging from the back of the cow, which was lying on the ground in the middle of all these blackberry thorns. So we had to get a tractor in with a device called a hiplifter attached to the front. Mook got the tractor into the blackberry bush and lifted the cow into a standing position. I quickly administered an epidural to stop her pushing and to numb the area.

Jandy and I then had to spend fifteen minutes cleaning the uterus off before we could set about pushing the thing back in. Now, to put this in perspective, imagine a potato sack filled with meat and you can start to imagine the size and weight of a uterus. Jandy had to take the weight of it while I tried to tuck the potato sack back into the cow. It's a hard physical job, holding this big slippery thing while applying gentle pressure to push a bit of it back in before re-adjusting to grasp the next bit of uterus and push that in. It requires a particular type of strength and endurance in the forearm muscles.

We got it in then used a special needle, a Buhner needle, to stitch the vulva shut. A Buhner needle is a fierce-looking implement: about 25 centimetres long with a large handle and a curved point that has a central hole in it to thread your stitching material through. You need to make sure your epidural is working well before you pierce the skin with such a formidable tool, running it up and down, parallel to the vulva, so the uterus doesn't fall out again.

We fixed the cow up pretty well and Mook lifted her right out of the blackberries and it was job done.

Our overalls were a bloody slimy mess and we changed out of them before jumping in the car to drive the 40 kilometres back to town to enjoy the rest of our Sunday. There had been rain recently and the countryside had a lovely green tinge to it that enhanced every aspect of rural life. The sun was poking its first rays over the small escarpment to the east of the Manilla–Barraba road, throwing light on the much taller, jagged range that jutted out of the landscape to the west. It looked like being a glorious day.

As we approached the outskirts of Barraba, dwarfed by massive old silos where the speed limit starts to drop, my phone began to rumble its cheery tune. When you're on call, your phone ringing is anything but cheery. There's a small part of you that hopes that it might just be someone you know ringing for a chat, or perhaps a wrong number. But who was I kidding at 7 a.m. on a Sunday? I looked at the screen and it was a Manilla number. I picked up. A horse had a badly cut leg at a property back out on the road we'd just come down – 20 kilometres past Mook's place. So we turned around and went back the way we came.

We arrived at the property on the green river flats, driving past a neat weatherboard cottage to what looked like the stable and yard areas. We found a tiny blonde girl covered in blood. She must have been only eight years old.

'Oh my God, are you okay?' I asked, wondering what we'd walked into here.

'Yeah, I'm okay but Rocket's not so good,' she said.

On closer inspection, we could see the whole yard was spattered like a forensic police drama. And there was the victim, a buck-skin quarter horse with a bloody bandage on its front right leg skulking in the corner.

'It was squirting blood so I got the bandage on,' the girl said.

'What's your name?'

'Rosie.'

'Okay, Rosie, you've done a fantastic job. You might have saved Rocket's life.'

'It's my horse so I wanted to help it.'

Rosie's mum was holding Rocket, who was twitching with nerves, but he let me approach and I got a sedative into him. I took the bandage off and saw that he had severed his digital artery. Horses' feet need a strong blood supply so the blood is pumped in under enormous pressure. If these digital arteries get severed, the blood can spray out for metres. And if Rosie hadn't got this bandage on, Rocket would likely have bled to death. I redid the bandage, packing it very firmly, and told the family to leave it on for about three days and Rocket should be fine.

By this stage it was well after breakfast time. Jandy and I had worked up an appetite. We drove the now 60 kilometres back to Barraba to refuel and get something to eat at the service station. But just as we pulled into the driveway, the cheery ringtone burbled again.

'Yeah, g'day, Duncan Thompson here. Barry's just eaten a bucket of 1080 fox bait.'

Barry was Duncan's red kelpie. 'Okay. That's not good,' I said. Normally the tiniest sniff of 1080 will kill a dog. 'Is he still breathing?'

'Yeah, he's right as rain at the moment.'

'How much of it did he actually eat?' I asked.

'He's eaten the whole bucket. I was putting out chicken heads. I had 'em in the front seat of the ute, but I left the window down slightly and the dog took a giant running jump and managed to get through. He ate the whole lot before I caught him.'

The way fox baiting works is that they inject the poison into the eyeballs of the chickens so the fox swallows the whole thing and is then killed when digestion begins.

'Gee, that doesn't sound promising. That's enough poison to kill him fifty times over. I'm not sure that we can do much but get him here as fast as you can; we might be able to ease his suffering.'

'All right, I'm on me way.' Duncan sounded pretty cut up about it. He really liked Barry.

I refuelled the car while Jandy went inside to buy us a pack of salt-and-vinegar chips each, then we raced over to the clinic to wait for Barry and Duncan. They were thirty minutes' drive away, and while I knew they'd be driving hard, I half-expected that we wouldn't even see them. Barry would probably die on the front seat of the car and Duncan would turn around to dig a hole back at home.

But the ute came screeching into our shed and Barry jumped out the door with his tail in the air and his nose down, sniffing at all the exotic animal smells that vet clinics provide. He was a proper working dog, thin and muscled with a shining coat.

'Are you sure he ate the bait?' I said. 'He should be dead by now.'

'I saw him polishing off the last of 'em,' Duncan said. 'Shoulda seen how guilty he looked. He knew he was going to get in big trouble but he'd obviously figured it was going to be worth it.'

'Okay.'

Vets have a bit of a party trick in this situation. There's a drug called apomorphine, a close friend of morphine, which has a little bit of the opioid sedative effects of morphine and a really exaggerated nausea effect. We can dissolve the tablet in water and inject it, or we can just take the tablet and pop it under the lower eyelid of the animal, where it absorbs really quickly. So I did that and Duncan looked at me strangely, just as people always do when you put it there. 'My dog needs to vomit,' they're thinking. 'Why are you putting something in his eye, you moron?' But before you've had time to finish explaining, the dog will be puking on the floor, and that's what Barry started to do. First one chicken head then another and another, till we had the whole finger-licking bucket load on the floor. He vomited up more chicken heads than I thought a dog could possibly swallow.

We stood there, still thinking Barry was going to drop dead at any moment, but he just stared back at us, wagging his tail and coming in for more pats from Duncan, who he must have noted was being unusually affectionate this day, especially considering he'd just swallowed all the guy's yummy chicken heads.

I went over and had a look at all the heads on the floor and noted that none of them had been chewed. Barry had just inhaled them.

'All I can think of, Duncan, is that even though your dog has eaten more 1080 than any dog in the history of poison, he hasn't absorbed any of it. Because he didn't chew any of the heads, the eyes are intact, so none of the poison got released.'

Then the phone rang. There was a difficult calving 60 kilometres down the road, out towards Narrabri. 'Duncan we've got to run. Ben's across the road and he'll keep an eye on Barry till I get back, but I'm pretty sure the little bugger's gotten away with it.' And so we left our satisfied customers and raced off to the calving.

It was pretty straightforward and we were back at the clinic less than two hours later. We had to hurry back though because we got a call that a kelpie with a branch sticking out its chest was waiting for us at the front door with its owner. The dog had impaled itself on the branch while jumping over a log. The stick had broken off and the owner had wisely left it there and rushed straight in. The poor thing could hardly breathe and was lucky to be alive. We rushed in to open the surgery. The first step was to get an IV line into him and some oxygen running, before knocking him out and starting the operation to remove the stick. There was no time to waste. The dog wasn't able to breathe on his own, so Jandy had to breathe for him by squeezing the reservoir bag on the anaesthetic machine, forcing air into the lungs.

I might have had the confidence of a full year's experience behind me but I was still a new vet and this kind of pressure was tough. I traced the stick deep into the abdomen. Luckily it had gone all that way without piercing any major organs. The only problem was that it had gone through the diaphragm and one of the lungs had collapsed. Access to the diaphragm is tricky. You're at the very margins of the abdomen and it is tucked right up under the rib cage. All I could hope for was that the hole was small and accessible, and that none of the structures that run through the diaphragm, like the oesophagus, were involved. I got lucky. When the stick was removed it left a nice neat hole that I could get to. I flushed and cleaned the hole, then started to stitch it closed.

'Now inflate the lungs and hold it until I tell you to let the air out,' I instructed Jandy. I needed her to pump the lungs up to expel as much of the extraneous air from the chest cavity as she could while I stitched up the last part of the hole.

'Okay, Jandy, ease off the bag. Time to see if he can breathe for himself.'

And he did. We seemed to be winning. I suppose we were on a bit of a high. What a day. It was barely lunchtime. But we'd pulled it off. Bad things come in threes, right, so we'd handled our quota, plus two more, and now we could get on with the weekend.

And that's when the cheery phone rang again. A snakebite on a dog. They were coming in. I dealt with that then the phone rang again with another calving. I called Ben to come in to recover the impaled kelpie and we left for the calving. But while we were on the 100-kilometre drive north towards Warialda, the phone rang again. It was another calving back east of Barraba. I told them we'd be late.

By 3 p.m., we'd almost reached Warialda when the darned phone rang again. I was starting to loathe that tinny electric sound.

It was another problem calving, 60 kilometres to the north-east of Barraba. 'You should try calling the vet in Inverell,' I said. 'It's a long drive for him but he might be able to come. I just *can-not* get there. I'm having the day from hell and I've got two other calvings booked in ahead of you.'

The Warialda calving went smoothly. So we changed out of our overalls and headed for the one east of Barraba. We arrived at a rambling farmhouse that had obviously started as a small cottage before the verandas had been enclosed, then a fibro extension added to one side, while a weatherboard room was tacked onto the other, before it grew an aluminium-clad tumour out the back.

The whole family came out to greet us. They were young by farming standards. The parents were in their late thirties and they had a team of tidy looking kids who wanted to be in the thick of it all.

The animal in question was a small, red shorthorn heifer – a female that hasn't yet had a calf. I put my hand in her and couldn't quite make out what I was feeling. The head was there all right, but the legs seemed to splay out to the side in a way I'd never felt before. Puzzled, I pushed my hand in further, straining to get it in, until suddenly I felt sausage-like loops of tissue.

Oh Cripes! Intestines! I've screwed this up something terrible. I've pushed too hard and gone right through the uterus and into the heifer's guts.

It was the most horrible sinking feeling in my tired and rumbling belly. I paused for a moment, my hand still inside the heifer up to my armpits, and I thought … and I thought … I thought as hard as my weary brain could manage.

Hang on, those intestines are tiny. That's not the mum's guts. They're the calf's intestines … schistosomus reflexus!

I wasn't certain. I'd never seen one of these before, but surely that's what it had to be.

I pulled my arm out and tried to explain it to the parents, Derek and Cat Tobin. 'Basically, when you're forming embryonically, you start off as spinal cord and nerve tissue. Your body folds out from that spine and comes around and meets back again at the midline. This is why you see a lot of midline deficits like hernias or cleft palates and things like that. It's a failure of that folding mechanism.'

Derek and Cat's expressions indicated that maybe I wasn't making it so clear.

I continued: 'If you look at yourself, you're a tube on legs. This calf's condition occurs when that tube is forming, instead of coming back and meeting in the middle to enclose all your insides, the fold goes the wrong way, so you're actually inside out. That's *schistosomus reflexus*. That's what I think we've got here. The calf in there has all its organs on the outside.'

'Ah, okay. So what do we do about it?' was the fair and reasonable question from Derek. The heifer's smallness added to the degree of difficulty. The calf had zero chance of survival. So I just had to get it out. I couldn't bring it out through the vagina and I couldn't get good enough access to cut it up. I was going to have to do a caesarean.

I prepped up for the operation, inserting the epidural and shaving the heifer's sides while Jandy held the torch in the darkened crush.

The heifer responded by throwing herself on the floor into a couple of inches of mud. It was so muddy in those yards that I was already wearing gumboots, not items pressed into action that often in Barraba. The recent rain, combined with the cattle trampling through, had cut the yards up badly, producing a quagmire. *This is hopeless. She's going to die.* I pushed on. The cow had at least thrown herself down with the left side up so I could get at the uterus without all the guts falling out. I had to cut a much larger hole in her side than normal because the calf was so misshapen, with stiff legs splayed in all directions.

The whole family gathered around to watch. Word had passed around about this freak calf. All four kids displayed a genuine enthusiasm for the world, so the prospect of seeing such a calf had them circling in hushed excitement. This was the best thing. They talked about it in terms of aliens and monsters. The flash of their camera periodically lit up my muddy little operating theatre.

As I cut into the uterus and opened it up, the first thing I saw was organs sitting out in the open, all attached to the calf's body but otherwise floating free in the uterus. I felt relief and satisfaction that my diagnosis was correct. Thank goodness I was paying attention at uni that day. Everybody crowded in to get a look. Meat and bones were sitting out in the open. The ribs were turned upwards like wings. Butterflied. They were all oohing and gasping. It was better than television.

The calf's bones were fused and abnormally formed, so even though it was very small, it was much harder to get out than the normal streamlined calf. I prised the uterine tissue open and started manipulating the limbs, at the same time holding the uterus in place while I got Jandy and Derek to pull the bits out.

Together we wrestled everything out of the big hole and laid it out for everyone to see. The kids' excitement made the whole thing extraordinary. They seemed really switched on and I did my best to answer the questions they asked. The three girls and a boy ranged in age from six to twelve so they each required an explanation of different complexity. They were such enthusiastic people that I was happy to do it, even though I was tired and hungry and we had another calving hanging over our heads. I didn't know if the people who'd rung at 3 p.m. still needed help.

While I was instructing the kids, Jandy was stitching up the skin of the heifer and cleaning up. I started to take stock. This was the eighth job of the day. We were running low on gear. I knelt down beside Jandy as she injected antibiotics and anti-inflammatories and I whispered: 'Don't throw the needles away.'

'What?'

'Keep the needles.'

'Why?'

'We've run out. The next calving is only 60 kilometres away. We're not going back to town before we go, and we don't have any more needles.'

As farmers know, you can reuse needles just fine, but it's not exactly the look you're going for – turning up with old Trusty Rusty, your faithful injecting tool.

After Jandy was done stitching, the heifer seemed to bounce back fine, despite the mud and trauma and the size of the hole in her belly. She had no right to survive but she did – Derek and Cat even sent me the photos to prove it.

It was after the kids' bedtime, so we said our goodbyes, unpeeled our overalls and got back in the car. One job to go. When we found some reception on the top of a rise, I rang to check that we were still needed, but the bars proved to be phantoms and no conversation could take place so we pushed on. I'd checked in with them about four hours earlier and they'd said then that they still wanted us to come. They hadn't been able to get the vet from Inverell.

We drove up the long driveway, over grids and past the shapes of large dark animals in the fringe of our beams. As we crossed another grid and drove up to the house, two men came out into the spot of our headlights with forlorn looks on their faces that said we were definitely still needed.

'We didn't think you were coming,' the younger man remarked.

'Well, I said I'd get here, I just couldn't guarantee which month it would be.'

They were a father and son who ran a big operation and were in the middle of generational change. The father owned the property but the son owned the cattle. He had bought a load of small heifers from a very well-known local stud. They were only fifteen months old, and one of them – this tiny, runty heifer – was calving already. A bull at the stud had found its way into her paddock and got her in calf at six months of age. She barely came to above my hip.

I put my hand inside her and felt a head the size of a normal calf's head. 'There's no way that's coming out the back end,' I said, but they looked at me like I wasn't telling them anything they didn't already know. 'We can either shoot her or we're doing a caesarean.'

By this stage I was half praying they'd reach for the ammo. It was 11 p.m. and I hadn't had breakfast yet. I'd been going since 5 a.m. I'd done umpteen procedures. Large animals. Small animals. I had three blunt needles in my car and a pea-soup fog in my head.

'All right, we'll do the caesarean,' the son said.

Aaarrgghh …

'Rightio, Jandy, let's go. You know the drill. We're going to get this thing out.' We had to make a huge cut in relation to the size of the animal. The calf was big and the cow was small. She wouldn't have weighed 250 kilograms, about half the weight of a normal cow. We did the caesarean by rote. In the end it was nothing remarkable other than we pulled out a good 40-kilogram calf and I had massive pins and needles in my thumb. When you do a lot of suturing in one day, the pressure of the needle-holders on the edge of your thumb causes the tingling, and the suture material cuts through the skin of the last knuckle on your little finger where it naturally nestles. I was spent.

'Jandy, you should stitch this one up.'

I was stuffed and it was a good opportunity for her to learn. The farmer was giddy with excitement; he got a live calf and his heifer was up and kicking. Usually if a calving is held up this long, the calf has no chance, but because this thing was so big and the mother so small, it had never made it into the birth canal so neither mother nor baby suffered too much distress.

Such little victories are the joy that this job brings, but the pleasure centres of my brain had closed for the day, like an airport shutting for fog. The hunger centre was still operating at full capacity, however, as we climbed out of our overalls and drove into the night. It was almost 1 a.m. when we got home. We'd been going for twenty hours. Aside from all the jobs, we'd driven 480 kilometres. Five and a half hours of the day had been spent in the car. We'd only had the pack of salt-and-vinegar chips and a vanilla malt milk drink.

I sent Jandy to the shower first – thank God I had her to help me that day, otherwise I don't think I would have made it – while I cracked a beer. It was only a light beer because I was still on call but its rich hops and malts exploded into my mouth like a super-flash boutique brew.

After Jandy finished in the shower, I got in and then returned to the kitchen for a closer search of my young-single-person refrigerator. Eureka! A barbecue chicken.

The pleasure centre reopened for business. The flavour of that skin lingers with me to this day as one of the finest things I've ever tasted. We destroyed the chicken, leaving only a pile of gnawed bones. A full tub of ice-cream was also soon emptied and licked clean.

We said goodnight and crawled into bed. It was getting up towards 2 a.m. and we had to be at work in five hours. I was still on call until 7 a.m. The tiredness went through to my bones, and if the phone had rung again that night, I don't think I would have pretended to be wide awake when I answered. Or, if I did, I might have done what I used to do with Mum and just fallen straight back to sleep.

WHERE'S WALLY?

Anthony

At Christmas 2006 Dad turned up at my place and said, 'Go to the back of the car, Anthony. There are two things in there. One of them is your Christmas present.'

I went around to have a look and there in a box on the back seat were two beautiful snub-nosed, black and brown puppies.

I turned to Dad, feeling every bit as excited as I had the day he brought Stuart and Wesley home. 'What are they?'

'Dobermans. When they're little they don't have that long face.'

These guys looked like Rottweilers.

Dad knew I'd been looking for a dog. I'd almost taken one after a caesarean on a beagle. I was going to pitch to the owner that I'd waive the fee for one of the puppies, but I had some neighbours who were horrible people. They'd threatened to shoot our other neighbour's dog if it so much as set a paw on their property. Beagles would be the worst breed to get because they would pick up a scent and just take off in pursuit, regardless of fences. So I pulled out of that. But Dad had a friend with a lovely Doberman bitch which had just had a litter.

I was on call that day and got a request to go to the clinic. I grabbed one of the puppies and took him in for a road test. This puppy was the quieter of the two and no sooner had we hit the road than he was asleep. I carried him into the clinic and he didn't seem fazed by anything. As soon as I put him on a towel in a cage he just went to sleep.

When I returned home, Dad was playing with the other puppy. He was a different kettle of sardines altogether: very active and into everything, super affectionate and constantly looking for attention. He only had tiny teeth and claws and his prime method of gaining attention was to use them.

So I had a dilemma – the sooky, quiet puppy or the outgoing, exuberant one. I had no doubt that the quieter pup would be easier to raise and train but my heart lay with the active fellow. I liked his outlook on life: be active and demand attention. He was like me. So I chose him and he turned out to be fantastic.

He didn't have a name, and my flatmates – Hef and Izzo – and I racked our brains trying to think of one. We were mad keen fans of the TV show *Entourage*. There's a character in it called Turtle who has a Rottweiler. Hef and I were watching it when Turtle came on screen with his dog and the idea came to me to name my puppy Turtle. It stuck.

To this day when I'm watching the show and one of the actors calls out 'Turtle', my dog's head comes up and he's ready for action.

We were living in a house on a property owned by Geoff Scarlett. The place wasn't set up for a dog, so for the first few weeks, I kept Turtle in the bath while I was at work. It was the only place I could think of where he wasn't going to wreck the interior. We hadn't paid a bond. My career was the bond. And living with those guys I felt both house and career were constantly under threat.

Turtle hated being put in the bath and would go absolutely berserk when he was left there. However, when I returned home everything was always quiet and he was usually sleeping on the blanket that I had left for him.

I spent countless hours training Turtle, as I was acutely aware of how dangerous these dogs could be. He was very food-motivated so it was easy to teach him the basics. The hardest thing to teach a dog is to reliably come back. I would make him aware that I had a pocket full of dog food, and all it required was a quick whistle and he'd be sitting by my feet looking for a reward.

We were lucky that we lived on a property, not so much because of Turtle's antics, but because we were surrounded by lots of different species. I knew what damage dogs could do to livestock, so I would sit outside with Turtle in the paddocks, calmly talking to him while the horses and cattle watched and sniffed him. The first couple of times I had to sit on him to stop him going for them, but before long he would wait with me, watching the animals and basically just wanting to be patted.

He was a great mate and still is.

We had a student intern, Emily, who came to work with us at the Berry clinic, so we offered her our spare room to stay in. The day she started she drove direct from Sydney in the morning, did the day's work, and then headed to our place to settle in. I had touch footy and tennis that night so I wasn't going home after work and neither were Izzo or Hef. I drew a map for Emily and told her that her bedroom was the last on the left at the end of the hall.

'Great, can I have a key?' she asked.

'We don't lock the house. We don't even have a key. There's only Turtle, but he's a big pussycat.'

'Oh, okay. All right. No problems.' Being a city kid, she seemed a bit put off by that but trundled off gamely. She was asleep by the time I got home.

Next morning I took myself off for a jog and didn't see her again until we were back at the clinic, where she seemed to have an urgent need to tell me about something. But she appeared wary. Suspicious even. She waited until Trish and Geoff were around to back her up before coming out with it.

'You and Izzo are fond of animals, are you?' she said, half-smiling, half-frowning.

'Well, yeah, we're vets aren't we? What's up?'

'When I arrived last night, I wasn't sure which house it was, so I drove past a couple of times. I didn't think it could be your place because, like, the front door was wide open. I could kind of understand you leaving the place unlocked but leaving the door wide open seemed a bit, like, seriously loose.'

'I didn't leave it open,' I said. 'It was probably Izzo. He *is* seriously loose.'

'Well, anyway, I got my bags and came in. I still didn't know if I had the right place, and as soon as I went through that door I really hoped I had the wrong address. There was horse shit all the way down the hallway. I'm like, "Oh my God, what have I got myself into here? What are these guys into?"'

I looked at Trish and Geoff with an expression that said, 'I don't know what she's talking about. She's mad.' And they looked at me with furrowed brows and almost embarrassed smiles as Emily continued her tale, skirting that fine line between telling a funny story and totally alienating her new boss and housemate whom she'd only known for a day. 'I called out but there was no answer so I came down the hallway and got to the kitchen. Then I heard a noise coming from a bedroom. I was so scared. I wanted to, like, grab a knife but that would have been a bit weird, since I didn't know whether or not I was the intruder. Anyway, I snuck up to the door and peeked around the corner and there, standing on the bed, was a Shetland pony ... and it was eating a pack of Tim Tams.'

I felt the laugh coming from deep down in my guts and was barely able to get the single word out: 'Wally!'

When I'd settled down sufficiently, I explained to Emily that Wally was the neighbour's hopelessly obese pony that roamed the street unhindered by fences and was much loved by all. Wally had learnt that if he banged on doors hard enough with his little hooves they would often open. They would often break as well but that's another story.

Emily was warming up to her story now: 'Well he was eating those Tim Tams one at a time, like he was having the best day of his life and he wanted it to last forever. When he saw me, he looked at me like, "Crap, you got me. I can't lie to you, I'm not really meant to be here."'

She told us that she shooed Wally out and cleaned up the mess. Luckily for her – and my career – the poo was confined to the tiles in the hall so it cleaned up pretty easily.

I rang Izzo at Gerringong and had him rolling on the floor when I told him. It took a while for his belly laughs to die down so I could ask him: 'Mate, what were you doing with the Tim Tams in your bedroom anyway?'

'I didn't have them in my bedroom.'

'Well, Wally was eating them standing on your bed.'

'They were on top of the microwave.' We realised that Wally had gone into the kitchen, identified the brown and white packet as a desirable food item, taken it off the microwave – which was well above his head height – and then identified Matt's bed as a comfortable place to consume said food.

'What I can't get over is that I could have slept in that bed without realising a horse had recently been eating Tim Tams in it.'

We eventually moved out of Geoff's place with my career still intact. I settled into a place in town. Turtle continued to be my constant companion. He used to come with me to the pub. We'd go running on the beach. He became quite well known around town. Sometimes people would come into the clinic and talk about their animals with absolute adoration. They would always qualify it with 'You must hear this all the time' and then go on about how Max/Molly/Rory was the best dog ever, never does anything wrong. Well Turtle was that dog. You only get one or two dogs like that in a lifetime and I got one straight off.

One day I noticed him scraping his backside on the ground. Most people think this is a sign of worms, and it can be, but more often it signals trouble with the dog's anal glands. They are two little scent glands that sit at the base of the rectum so that when the dog passes faeces, it leaves its signature scent on each parcel. When dogs smell each others' bottoms, they're smelling that scent. It's like swapping business cards.

But a lot of dogs have problems with their anal glands, probably because they are eating a more processed diet than they would have had in the wild. Fixing the gland is not complicated, but it is one of the more disgusting jobs a vet has to face. The secretion from the gland is the vilest substance you can imagine. It stinks its own world of salty foulness. It's every bit as bad as a rotten calving except it's distilled into this tiny bundle of intensity, ready to squirt at you at any moment.

To clear the secretion and relieve the pain, you need to 'digitally express' the two anal glands, which means you put a glove on and stick your finger up the dog's bottom. The secretion shoots out through the hole. You only do it with your mouth open once.

Despite my many offers to teach clients to do it themselves, I haven't had a taker yet.

I figured that since I was a vet, I'd better get in and fix Turtle's glands myself.

Now, one of the great teachers at uni, Paul Hopwood, gave lectures like they were masterpieces; flowing from one subject to another, weaving his way through stories to make insanely boring subjects interesting. But he'd also single you out if he didn't like you and make a fool of you in front of everyone by asking difficult questions. So you'd sit there in a high state of anxiety praying that you weren't going to be picked on. I remember one day he said, 'Ladies and gentlemen, Australia's finest, what is the first thing you will feel when you stick your finger into a dog's bottom?'

I was sitting there thinking, 'Crikey, please don't pick on me. Is it the internal rectal sheaf? Is it the colon? Faeces? Is it some muscle? It could be anything. Please don't ask me.'

'Ladies and gentlemen, the first thing that you will feel when you stick your finger into a dog's bottom is the dog's jaws clamping around your wrist. Make sure someone is holding the dog's head firmly.'

I knew this, but not having anyone to hold Turtle's head I figured I'd just tie him up. I secured his head to a rail in the backyard at home with a really short and tight rope. He could sway around with his bum but if I kept a hold of his tail it should be all right. So, in the privacy of my own backyard, I began the process of performing this completely legitimate veterinary procedure – with my mouth firmly closed because I'd already filled my lifetime quota of mouth-open anal gland expressions. With my finger up Turtle's bottom I saw the balding dome of my new neighbour, Pete Godfrey, appear above the timber fence. Our eyes met. He looked at me and I looked at him.

I could read the good family man's thoughts.

'Mate, I'm a vet. I promise you,' I said. But it's hard to talk with your mouth firmly shut.

'Yeah … okay … ummm.'

We smoothed things over, but I think Pete's remained a little suspicious of me ever since.

PARVOVIRUS AND PROLAPSES

James

The sun was shining and the heat was already building at 7 a.m. when I arrived to open the Manilla clinic. The smell hit me before I'd even got the key into the lock. And even if I was able to overlook what lay inside – as if I'd be able to – I'd never forget that stench. It was the smell of economic disadvantage. Three dogs with parvovirus.

Barraba, Manilla and Bingara were triple-speed kinds of places. There were farms that were big, serious agricultural enterprises. Their sons had often returned from boarding schools and they also had three or four men working on them. One place had twenty stockmen running 11,000 breeding cattle. Then there were the smaller farmers who did it a lot tougher, working largely by themselves. Most of the properties around Manilla were soldier-settler kind of blocks – around 500 hectares. Big enough to offer a dream but small enough to consistently break hearts. You could run 150 or 200 cows on some of them but to make a good living you needed to run at least 300 breeders. A lot of those people scraped by, but they were on the edge.

And then there were the townies. When I arrived, Manilla was largely a welfare town. There were some rough people in the mix. It's four and a half hours from Sydney with affordable farming land, so a lot of tree-change types were also moving in. They injected life and money into the town, a trend which has accelerated since, but a decade ago we were still seeing a lot of animal diseases you associate with poverty. The most obvious of those was parvovirus in dogs.

Parvovirus is easily preventable with a vaccine, so it's virtually unheard of in affluent areas, but in poorer places people don't always follow the prompts. The victims are usually pups, about four to five months of age. They come in pale and flat. You lift their gums and there is no colour, but there's a lot of drool and perhaps the residue of vomit. Where there should be a bubbly, inquisitive puppy, you have a still, floppy and cold animal. And then the diarrhoea starts. It's got this awful odour because their intestinal lining is dying, rotting and coming away. It's a lot like Ebola for dogs; they poo themselves to death and die from dehydration.

It's a really heartbreaking thing to treat because the disease is entirely preventable, and the people who can't afford to get their dogs vaccinated also can't afford to treat them. It takes a huge amount of nursing support in unpleasant conditions. I know of clinics where if you walk in the door with a parvo dog, they say: 'If you want it treated, you've got to pay $1000 now, up front, otherwise we'll have to put it down.' Without treatment, they will almost always die.

The outbreaks tend to happen in the warmer months. Often after rain. And so it was that we found ourselves in a late-summer outbreak with three puppies in care. When I opened up that morning I had to go around, gagging, opening every door in the shed, but I knew we would be stuck with the smell for weeks. We had to keep the pups isolated because parvovirus is highly contagious, so we'd built a big cage out in a corridor separate from the other dogs. Their poo drained straight into a hole at the bottom. I had to put a gown and gloves on for quarantine purposes before I could pick them up, wipe them clean and hose out the cage. The pups had a miserable hangdog look. But I knew if Suzanne and I could keep them alive for a week that they'd live.

I disinfected everything and put them back in, knowing we'd be repeating the process soon enough. The dogs crapped on themselves all the time because they were so weak and couldn't get away from it. Then they got skin irritations and scalding from the poo. Suzanne and I would both clean them up, but she took most of that burden because I had to maintain infection control in case I had to handle other puppies during the day. That was my story, anyway, and I stuck to it. In a clinic with a few vets, the person dealing with the parvo dog wouldn't see any other puppies for the day, but we didn't have that luxury.

It grew hotter and smellier in the clinic and the warmth gave the odour an added pungency. I wasn't too displeased to be called out to a prolapsed rectum. I drove upstream along the Namoi River and turned left over a shallow crossing.

The farmer, Sean Reynolds, greeted me with a fluffy white Maltese faithfully at his heel.

'How old's the dog?' I asked, worried about the risk of giving it parvovirus.

'Lulu's about nine,' he said.

'Should be fairly safe from parvo, then.' The truth was that while I didn't know Lulu's exact age, I knew she had to be reasonably old because she was one of the most famous dogs in the district. A few years earlier, before my time, Sean had been out walking a sheep paddock with Lulu trotting about nearby when he heard a commotion behind him. He'd spun around to see Lulu being lifted into the air by giant dark wings. A wedge-tailed eagle had swooped in and picked up the dog, presumably mistaking her for a small lamb. He saw Lulu get carried away beyond the treeline, yacking and squealing.

Sean rang the clinic, heartbroken, asking that if anybody notified us about a badly beaten-up dog, or if they saw one falling from the heavens, to call him.

And sure enough, a neighbour soon turned up at the clinic with Lulu, who was carrying a few cuts and scratches but was otherwise unharmed. Presumably the wedgie got the shock of its life when the meek little lamb it had picked up for dinner suddenly sprouted canines and started using them.

Sean showed me to the prolapsed cow. This one had a prolapsed rectum, where the colon turns itself inside out and protrudes out the rear of the cow. Now, the usual treatment for this would be to push it back in and do a purse-string stitch to tighten the anus, leaving the animal enough room to defecate but hopefully not enough for its bum to fall out again.

Unfortunately, the cow in question here had been running around for a long time with this thing hanging out before Sean had noticed it. The exposed flesh had become filthy and started to die off in places. I didn't think I could put it back inside her without risking serious side effects.

So I called Ben and explained the situation. He thought about it for while. 'Well, there is another technique you could use ...' and he proceeded to tell me of a method we certainly weren't taught at university. It sounded so far-fetched I thought he was pulling my leg.

'Are you for real?' I asked.

'Yeah, yeah. It's a great technique. Great technique.' As usual, he was very excited and I really had to trust his sincerity.

So I went over to Sean and explained that I was about to make his cow a prosthetic backside and could he please find me a piece of polypipe. He looked at me like I was some kind of wild cowboy. But he came back with a metre of black irrigation pipe.

I took a look. 'Nah, can you maybe get us a slightly wider bit? Maybe two inches.' He went off again with the famous dog never far behind. By the time he came back with the right-sized pipe, I'd given the cow an epidural and was ready to begin. The prolapse was protruding 15 centimetres out the back, so I cut off a 30-centimetre piece of pipe.

Remembering Ben's instructions, I drilled a couple of holes halfway along the pipe from one side to the other, but not directly through the middle – they were off to the side about one-third of the width.

I took the pipe and eased it into the prolapsed rectum so that half of the pipe was inside the cow and half outside, but all of that outside portion was covered by the prolapsed rectal tissue. I picked up a needle and thread and stitched the pipe to the rectum through the pre-drilled holes, conveniently aligned just on the outside of the cow. I then rummaged through my box of goodies and pulled out some Penrose drain, which is a flat white piece of rubber tubing designed to drain wounds after surgery. It looks a bit like a tapeworm, and in a bush practice like ours we find it comes in very handy as a tourniquet. And that's how I was going to use it here.

I tied the Penrose drain as tight as I could around the pipe, hard up against the normal skin. A rubber tourniquet cuts off the blood supply to the tissue, so if you wanted to be technical about it you might call it a rectal prolapse amputation. It does its work over a week or two, amputating the external part and forming a scar, joining up the skin with the part of the rectum that used to be 15 centimetres inside the cow but which is now flush with the anus. Excuse the pun. So in effect, it performs the cutting and stitching procedure all by itself, meanwhile the cow is able to relieve itself through the pipe.

'Couple of weeks later, no one would ever know it was there,' Ben had said on the phone. 'Never know. Never know it was there. Great technique. Great technique.'

'But how do we remove it?' I'd asked him.

'You don't. You put the stitches that attach it to the animal on the outside of the Penrose drain so that when the prolapse dies away, there is nothing holding it in place any more and it just falls out with the next defecation.'

Now I could actually see it in place I could appreciate the true elegance of this solution: the pure genius of my predecessors in bush vetting.

'How's it going to shit?' Sean wanted to know.

'Out the polypipe. You've just got to feed it wet feed. I wouldn't stand behind it though. I reckon it would have a lethal range.'

He came out with a camera and started taking photos, though I think they all came out blurred. He was laughing too hard to hold the thing steady. Especially with the money shot when it pooed.

RAMPAGING RAMBO

Anthony

The first job booked in for the Tuesday run out to Shoalhaven Heads was to euthanase an aggressive dog. That always raises the question of, 'What's it going to do to me when I'm trying to shuffle it off this mortal coil?'

I turned up at the address on River Road near the Heads Hotel with these misgivings rumbling away at the back of my mind. A ute was parked out the front with a big aerial, oversized bull bar, cages on the back, Bundaberg Run and Rum Pig stickers, the full I'm-a-wild-man-in-suburbia catastrophe.

A lot of growling and woofing was coming from out the back.

'Oh, yeah. You're the vet, are ya?' said the bloke advancing towards me. It seemed like he didn't believe I was a vet. I was driving a Magna and looked fourteen.

'Yep. That's me.'

'G'day. Shane.'

'Yeah, hi. I'm Anthony.'

Shane shook hands like he meant it. He might have been thirty but looked older, rougher – unshaven, no shoes, tattoos and boardies.

'Rambo's out the back.' He walked me through towards the deep-throated barking. 'Mate, I don't want to put the dog down but the missus says it's either her or the dog. She won in a toss-up.' He shot me a grin that said he may, or may not, have been joking. 'She reckons they're dangerous around the kids, but he's never bitten anyone. He growls a bit when the kids run around, but he's only playing. He hates intruders, though; a bloke came over the back fence after a night at the pub and he left minus a thong and a piece of his jeans. He won't be comin' back.'

We walked into the backyard which was messy with toys and swings and clothes hanging from the line. There were other dogs there yapping away, but I didn't pay attention to them. Because there was Rambo, just looking at me. Dogs that are truly threatening do not need to bark. Barking is a sign of fear. Rambo didn't know fear.

My response was to puff my chest out and pretend that I didn't know fear either. I don't think he bought it.

Rambo was a bull Arab, an Australian breed crossed to have the speed and stamina to catch a feral boar, and the size and ferocity to take it down. *Holy moly! You've got a dog like this in here with the kids.* They are trained to catch and rip the throats out of pigs, which aren't hugely different in a dog's eyes from a three-year-old child. Kids are pink, they squeal a lot, they move at high speed and don't have a lot of respect for dogs. *You're an imbecile for letting it walk around with the toddler.*

I'd argue that these sorts of dogs don't even have a place in towns, let alone children's backyards. The writing was on the wall for Rambo. He had attacked intruders and he was growling at the kids. Being a dog that was bred and trained to kill, I felt he was on a natural progression. It wasn't his fault, but the next stop was going to be the six o'clock news.

'Okay, mate, you'll have to give me a hand here because I'm on my own. Can you hold up a vein and I'll give her the injection to put her to sleep and away we'll go.'

'I can't, mate,' he said, still carrying himself like the tough guy that nothing could trouble. See m'ute. See m'dogs. See me.

'Well, you're going to have to because I'm here on my own. It's your dog and you want to put her down so you'll have to help.'

'Nup … can't,' Shane said.

'Why?'

Tears started to form in his eyes and the façade crumbled.

'I can't do it, mate. I can't. Not to Rambo.' He was backing away.

Shivers. What am I going to do? I didn't even have a muzzle. I needed another vet.

'Okay, I'll have to take the dog back to Berry where I've got someone to help me. But I've got to do my house calls around the Heads first and I don't think Rambo would be so welcome. I'll give him some sedation now and come back and get him when I'm done. Hopefully he'll be nice and calm by the time I get back.'

I raced out to the car. *What am I going to give this dog?* I rummaged around through my boxes and couldn't find anything appropriate. I went into the Esky and found some horse tranquiliser. *Oh well, that's all I've got.*

I drew up the syringe and took it back to the yard. 'You're going to have to hold Rambo for this injection, otherwise I can't help you, but don't worry, we're not killing him now, we're just relaxing him.'

I shoved the needle into Rambo's front leg and as soon as I finished I jumped back, but Shane was holding him firm and he was fine.

Leaving them there, I went to do my rounds, patting the white fluffy dogs and the overweight cats of our mostly elderly clients, all the while dreading this thing waiting for me at the end, hoping the dog was comatose by the time I returned. My rounds were fairly quick that day and I got back to find Rambo patrolling the yard, no more chilled than before. If anything, he looked like he'd had a couple of beers and was ready for a blue.

My heart sank. I only had the Magna, hardly the aggressive-animal transport vehicle of choice. But I made some room on the back seat and gave Shane a leash to put on Rambo's collar. I opened the back door and Shane, who had rebuilt his tough-guy front in my absence, helped him into the car.

Rambo was so tall his head touched the roof, forcing him to lean forward over the front seat. Shane took the opportunity to tie the leash to the passenger-side head rest. He gave Rambo a pat on the head, ruffled his ears. 'All right, mate. I'll be seein' ya.' He didn't want to talk to the dog or me. I suspect it was to disguise the fact he was crying. It was kind of touching, but I wasn't feeling his pain. This dog was a ticking time bomb. To be unable to handle the inevitable results of that stupidity and then to dish it off to someone else was quite galling. I wasn't feeling at my most empathetic. But at least he'd had the decency to call a vet.

I drove back to Berry hunched into the wheel because Rambo was leaning over my shoulder, his foul breath caressing my cheek as his panting lengthened and deepened. The sedation was kicking in.

Arriving at the back of the clinic, I was relieved it had all gone smoothly. He hadn't eaten my ears, for example. But I had to lean in with my face next to his slobbering jowls to untie him and that took a few deep breaths and a puff of the chest. Again, however, Rambo remained calm.

Both Geoffs were there and I knew that with their great experience they'd be able to help me. Just as I walked through the door, though, the phone rang. It was a specialist in Sydney returning a call I'd made earlier. I really had to take this call. Specialists are busy people who have taken the time to help for little return.

Geoff Manning was at the door as I brought Rambo in. 'Geoff, this is the dog that needs to be put down. Can you do it for me? I've got to take this call from the specialist.'

'Yep. I've got it.'

It was a long call and by the time I got off the phone, it was about 3 p.m. and the two Geoffs had gone. I presumed Rambo had been dealt with, and I was going about some other jobs when I heard a strange noise from the internal laundry. *What's that?* I looked in through the door and there was Rambo tied up in the shower recess, alive. *What the heck is going on?*

Rambo seemed keen to know what the heck was going on too. He looked cranky and distinctly un-sedated now. *Why didn't they put him down when they had the chance?* I couldn't go in and get him. To do that, I'd have to untie him, exposing myself with no help if things got ugly.

I was fuming. There was nothing I could do but call Geoff Manning and get him to come back to the clinic. He explained that they had both been called to different jobs at the same time and had had to leave immediately. He offered to come back in and help me with Rambo while the sedation was still working.

But it was too late. No one was going anywhere near this dog now. The nurse, Marie, and I tried wrapping sedatives in wet dog biscuits and sliding the bowl towards him with a long-handled broom, but he just looked at the food with no interest.

I pulled out a marker pen and a piece of printer paper and wrote: 'DO NOT ENTER THIS ROOM. AGGRESSIVE DOG.'

I went about the rest of my afternoon work, seeing clients for the usual round of vaccinations and tests, and then I got to work stitching-up a kelpie called Ronald that had torn his leg on a barbed-wire fence. It was all quite routine but I was engrossed in the procedure when I sensed a movement out of the corner of my eye. I looked up but nothing was there. That was odd. Marie had just left my side, but I could hear her out the front talking to a customer with a yapping lap dog joining in the conversation. Then I saw the flash again, clearer now. It was

Rambo, the 80-kilogram killing machine; prowling the practice, his hunter's nose close to the floor.

Suddenly, the clinic had a new owner.

He came right up to me, sniffing around. His back was the height of the table I was operating on. Rambo was hungry and perhaps even scared, so anything could have happened.

I was sterile for the procedure in hand, in my green surgical gown with a white mask and light blue hat, so I couldn't touch anything outside of the sterile surgical field. When you're operating you need a nurse to do everything for you: turn the anaesthetic up or down; wipe your brow.

And then Rambo headed for the door.

Crikey! What about that dog yapping in the waiting room. Rambo's gunna make a beeline for him. He'll have killed Fluffy and chewed the owner's arm off before we can even blink.

'Marie. Close the door,' I shouted, as loud as I could without sounding like a madman.

I think she realised the problem and quickly closed it. I tried to follow the dog with my sterile gloved hands in the air. He wandered into the cage and did the biggest poo I'd ever seen. It had to be 30 centimetres long. Then he just wandered past me like I didn't exist and into the sterile surgery, where the kelpie was lying anaesthetised on the table.

He's gunna smell blood and jump on the table and eat Ronald.

Not wanting to startle Rambo, I steadily waved my hands in the air and coaxed him out of the surgery. Somewhat luckily, he turned back into the laundry, at which point I broke with sterility protocols and slammed the door shut.

It turned out Marie had gone into the laundry to get something but had left the door ajar. Rambo had then slipped his collar and was free. I wrote another note, bigger and bolder this time, and said to Marie that if she set foot inside that room again it was going to be her job to euthanase the bloody dog. There's a line in the movie *The Grand Budapest Hotel* where the ever-cool Gustave says that 'rudeness is merely an expression of fear'. And if I was a bit short with Marie it was definitely a product of the dread I felt having this creature in the practice.

By the time Geoff arrived back at the clinic Rambo was wide awake, hungover and very pissed off. And if Geoff copped a further expression of my fear – 'Geoff, where have you been? This is a disaster!' – it might have had something to do with the guttural growls now emanating from the shower recess.

Geoff explained that he'd had a rotten calving that took a while to get out, and I gave him a rundown of the fun afternoon we'd been having. 'So we've got this ridiculous situation and I don't know how we can handle it. The dog's got no collar, no muzzle, he's free. How are we going to do it?'

He looked at me with just a hint of a smile. 'Have you got a cow halter in your car?'

'Yeah.'

'Good. Go and get it and I'll show you what we're going to do.'

I went and got the halter and brought it back in.

Geoff took a look at it. 'That oughta do. Right, when I tell you, open the door a little bit.' He moved over behind the door. 'Okay, now. Open it! Just a bit.'

I turned the handled and opened the door and Rambo stuck his head out. Geoff quickly put the cow halter over his snout and tightened.

The dog now had Geoff attached to it. Geoff still smelt like a rotten calving, which I was quite pleased about because Rambo took an interest in Geoff, nuzzling into his arms and appearing quite friendly.

'I think he likes you,' I said. 'Diced and chewed and washed down with a few dog biscuits and a glass of Chianti.'

'I think I should have washed a bit more thoroughly before coming back,' he said, with Rambo licking his forearm. 'Now go and draw up any and all of the sedatives that you can think of in a very large volume because we're going to get one chance to sedate this dog and it better work.'

So I went and drew up horse sedatives, horse anaesthetics, dog sedatives, cow sedatives. Everything in one big needle. One super sleepy cocktail. One thing I didn't have in it was Lethabarb, the euthanasia drug. You need an IV in his front leg for that. I didn't think Rambo would be keen to let me shave a nice little rectangle on his front leg then hunt around for a vein. He would have had my face first. And I knew from personal experience that the Lethabarb needle stung a lot if you missed the vein.

'How are we going to get this stuff into him?' I asked. 'He's gunna tear us apart if I hit it with a needle.'

'Look, I think he is going to be okay. I'll just talk to him and give him a pat and you be quick.' I bowed to Geoff's experience, but I was dubious. It was cool in the clinic yet I seemed to be sweating a lot. Despite his calm exterior, Geoff looked pretty sweaty too.

'Okay, as long as you're at the bitey end, I'll be at the smelly end.'

After a cascade of screw-ups, it seemed miraculous that the plan worked perfectly. Then Geoff took Rambo out the back and walked him around like he was a pet. Eventually Rambo started to wobble. He lay down and his eyes rolled back into his head and he fell into a comatose state. We still had to get the Lethabarb in so I clipped his fur and put a muzzle on him. And even as we did that, despite the massive amount of sedation coursing through his veins, he continued a deep, guttural growl, baring his teeth right up to the gums. Fighting in his dreams.

Normally you line up a needle with your head close to the barrel of the needle and parallel to the vein, much like using a pool cue. On this occasion I didn't want my face anywhere near Rambo and managed to successfully give the injection from about a metre away. Rambo uttered a final, feeble growl and passed away peacefully. It was only then that the sadness hit me. A great surge of pity for Rambo welled up inside. It wasn't his fault. He'd been the wrong dog in the wrong place and unfortunately had to pay for the irresponsible decisions of his owner.

A WELSH OF EXPERIENCE

James

After about eighteen months in Barraba and Manilla, my thoughts started to turn towards what came next. I got on very well with my boss, Ben. He was a great mentor and friend. He taught me a lot and I enjoyed his company. We had a chat one day and he broached the subject for me, asking what I wanted to do in the future.

'I'm thinking about going overseas and doing the locum-UK thing,' I said. 'But I'm not sure.' Going to Britain is a well-trodden path for vets, who can pick up high-paying temporary jobs while getting a chance to see a bit of the world.

'Okay, that sounds good,' he said. 'It's something that I always wished I did but it never worked out for me. I was always on the way there but never quite got the chance to leave.' There was a hint of regret in his voice, before he perked up: 'But if you stay then there's the potential to buy into this business.'

I had a real fork-in-the-road decision to make. Business was going well, particularly in Manilla where it was growing, so it could have been a lucrative move to buy in. I loved the job and loved the people. I was really happy. I'd learnt a lot there that I would never have got a chance to learn at a high-end practice in Sydney, where people want the most experienced guy with the big reputation operating on their little Trixiebelle. People had no money in Manilla and Ben was happy for us to give complicated surgeries a crack for a smaller fee: removing foreign bodies; dogs hit by cars; snakebites. I'd done all these dramatic things, but I'd never travelled much. I was keen to see the world. So I had to make that decision. Once again I over-thought it and lost a lot of sleep. Owning my own practice or a share in one was definitely what I wanted to do with my life. But I was single and carefree and it seemed like now was the time to explore the world.

About a week later, Ben and I were out the front packing his car to go to a job when he looked up from the door. 'Have you thought more about what you want to do?'

'Yeah, I have. I think I'm going to go travelling.'

He was great about it. He appreciated that it was not about the money. 'It's something I didn't get to do in my career,' he repeated.

After two years in Barraba and Manilla, I suddenly found myself arriving in London with a big pack on my back and a small one on my front, carrying all the stuff I needed to start a new life. In true tightwad backpacker fashion, I'd saved $150 by opting for a thirteen-hour stopover in Kuala Lumpur, and now, exhausted, I was booked into a six-quid-a-night backpacker dormitory. Not even my sixteen roommates could wake me for those first fourteen hours. The enormous hostel was called the Generator. It was in a converted electricity substation and slept about 2000 other tightwad partying youth. So I had a very good time.

It was hard to move out of the hostel because you'd go out till 4 a.m., sleep in and miss the cut-off for checking out. So you'd end up doing the same thing the next night, as it only cost six quid to stay on. And I had to remain in London for a week anyway, until I had an appointment at the Royal College of Veterinary Surgeons to be sworn in as a vet.

I got a cab to their little office in Chelsea suffering severe 'lifestyle fatigue'. I had to fill in a lot of forms that were hard to focus on. It sent my mind racing back to university when a lecturer had once posed us the hypothetical question: 'If you were faced with the choice of saving a baby or a dog, which one would you save?' No one chose the dog. 'Well you're not allowed to work in the UK,' he said, 'because their oath requires you to put the animal first.' So I might have had my fingers crossed while I swore the RCVS oath. I just needed to get back out into the fresh air.

Part of the reason Britain was so attractive to young Australian vets was that the locum rate was £180 a day. That equated to about AUD$450 back then. The locum agencies had long lists of available jobs. You could pick and choose because there was a shortage of vets and Australian locums were in demand. I think of Australians as laid-back and perhaps a little idle, but over there we were known for how hard we worked.

I went through the long job list and saw that there was one in northern Wales. That sounded interesting. A lot of people in northern Wales still spoke Welsh as their first language. It was a genuine enclave of isolated farmers who were fiercely proud and vociferously hated the English. *That's what I'm looking for. A bit of an experience wider than drinking Foster's in a youth hostel.*

I put in an application and soon after, while I was wandering along the road out the front of the British Museum getting a rare dose of culture, I received a call from the practitioners, a husband-and-wife team, John and Caroline Evans.

'Hello James,' a cheery voice chirped over the phone in an accent that I hadn't much heard before, but with which I would become very familiar. We chatted on the phone as cabs and busses whirled by then John offered me the job. 'Great, I'll see you there in two weeks.'

I set my alarms sufficiently early to escape the Generator and travelled north, where I hooked up with some mates, Nick and Alice, who were doing the same thing in Yorkshire as I was doing in Wales. We carried on around the dales and moors where the famous vet and writer James Herriott had practised, and had a great time soaking it all in. And then it was onto the train for Wales.

I could see long before I got there that I was in for a visual treat. Impossibly green hills and picture-book farms rose up to the left of the train and, to the right, the Irish Sea drifted away into a blue haze. My new boss, John Evans, was waiting for me at the nearby Colwyn Bay railway station. He piled all my things into his car and took me to the clinic, giving me the rundown as we went.

John was Welsh, had grown up in north Wales and spoke Welsh, he said. He'd met Caroline at university in Liverpool. They'd married and set up practice in Abergele, but her being English made life difficult for her.

We drove under the North Wales Expressway and he pointed up ahead to the huge mountains looming in front of us to the right. 'That's Snowdonia and Mount Snowdon is over there behind those clouds.'

I was suitably impressed.

Abergele, population 10,000, wasn't the prettiest town, nestled in behind the motorway as it was. But it was Wales! There were castles on the hilltops. (I'd even end up being mates with a guy who lived in one. A group of us went over there for beers and he had an inflatable adventure course inside the walls. It was wild.)

'Our clinic is called the Bryn Vet Surgery,' John said after we'd passed through the centre of town and started up a steep incline. 'Bryn means "hill" in Welsh.' Good name for it, I thought. He explained that I was replacing a female vet who'd been bitten by an Akita, a Japanese fighting dog, and who had lost the use of her arm as a result.

We pulled up at a beautiful old three-storey house just outside town. The bottom floor was the clinic. The staff rooms were on part of the second floor and then I had the remainder of the second floor plus the third floor and the attic to call home. The deal as a locum, on top of the generous wage, was that I also got accommodation and a car. The digs were great, very roomy for one bloke. The car, a beaten-up Rover, was less impressive.

It was wonderful, however, to have arrived after having spent the better part of a month travelling around. I remember going to the supermarket, Tesco, and buying a big load of groceries to set myself up. It was all exciting. All the brands were new and the packaging different. I settled into my flat on that first afternoon and made myself an extravagant meat-and-three-veg dinner. I'm not the best cook so I kept it simple and just amped up the spices and sauces. Then, with a full belly and a sense of adventure I wandered down the hill, long after dark at 5.30 p.m.

Town was about a mile away. I stuck my head into the first pub I came to, The Bull. It was quiet and a little seedy. I had a beer there. Not much going on. So I wandered around the corner to a pub that I'd seen on my way to Tesco, The Bee, which I deduced from the signs was famous for carrying on the ancient Welsh tradition of karaoke. But all was quiet there too, so I started to venture back towards the clinic, skipping a quiet-looking pub called the Harp along the way and ducking out of the cold night air into the George and Dragon. It was a very old pub, probably Georgian era. I walked into the crowded bar and ordered a beer. The motherly woman behind the counter whose name I later learnt was Mary Lynham looked at me inquisitively.

'Ooooo, where are you from, dear?'

'Australia.'

'Heeeeee's from Australia,' she announced to the rest of the pub. The word rippled around the packed bar. The guy next to me looked me up and down. 'Australian, eh? Do you play cricket?'

'Yeah.'

'Great. We've got training tomorrow. Where are you staying?'

'At the vet clinic.'

'Great. I'll pick you up at 9 a.m. and take you. There's two other Australians in Abergele and they both play – but I have to say that they're pretty shit by Australian standards; they go okay in Wales, though. I'll introduce you. I've got to go but I'll see you tomorrow.'

Then a girl came over. 'What part of Australia are you from? I travelled around Australia last year. Come over and have a beer.'

There was a table of about a dozen people of a similar age to me. I started chatting to them and more kept coming in. There were soon twenty people there. A lot of them had been to Australia so we had a lot to catch up on. What was fascinating to me was that all their parents were on the other side of the pub drinking with their own generation.

There was a real family feel to the pub that I'd never experienced before. I'd be chatting to some bloke and then his daughter would join us, then his father. The George and Dragon became a hub of my Welsh existence. These families were to become like second families to me. But all that was still ahead.

On Monday morning I looked out the window, ready to start my new job, and I couldn't get over how green and beautiful everything was. It was late February, so the days were still very short but there was just a hint of spring touching the glistening earth. Everything was wet.

As a vet, it's an enormous transition to go to a different country. Things have different names. They do things differently. So you're like a new grad again. You don't know the name of the drug you want. You're saying Clavulox and they're looking at you like you're mental because it's called Synulox over there. When they spay cats they go through the flank as opposed to the midline, where we do them in Australia. They use different suture patterns to stitch things up. It's important as the outsider to fit in and learn their ways.

Two years out of uni was a good time to do it. By the end of my time in Barraba I'd started to get comfortable. I had a bit of experience,

I knew what I was doing, and the clients knew me, so it all got a lot easier. I needed a real mind shift. While I had my way of doing things from Barraba, I wasn't too set in my ways to re-learn. And so I learnt a lot. They had more advanced equipment than Barraba. Things like small-animal ultrasound machines. And the large-animal side was different too. Instead of having graziers with 300 or 3000 cows, their farmers had only a handful of animals which were more intensively looked after – and they usually had names.

The horses and cows were different breeds. Some of the horses were huge; Shires were seventeen or eighteen hands. You needed a stepladder to give them an IV injection when they had colic. It was a very different kind of practice. Everything was new, fresh, exciting and scary.

Caroline handled the small-animal side of things. She was very serious, methodical and organised. Everything she did was professional and conscientious. I learnt a lot from her.

John was a funny bloke. We spent a lot of our time laughing. And John spent a lot of his time in trouble with Caroline for being disorganised and laid-back. They were a chalk-and-cheese kind of couple, which made them a great combination to work for. I'd often go to their place for dinner and hang out with their kids. They were really welcoming and they looked after me. But I worked very hard for them too.

One of my first jobs was to see to some sick calves in a barn for a farmer by the name of Mr Evans. All the cows were in barns in February. I'd drive around and wonder where all the animals had gone. But it was so wet and cold that the animals were inside because, for one, they do much better being warm in the barn, but also because if they were out on grass they'd destroy it by pugging it up into mud. But the downside of being in a barn was that, by the end of winter, they often

171

developed respiratory-tract infections and other diseases. And they were just sick of being cooped up. They wanted to get outside and eat some grass.

Pulling up at the farm, the first task was to locate the farmer, which could at times be a challenge. Some of these sheds were modern, like the type of iron sheds you'd find in Australia, but Mr Evans had one of the sheds that I loved. It was ancient, made of stone and with a very low ceiling and exposed beams. It was built at a time when people weren't as tall as they are now, so all of the doors were tiny (maybe this is why I liked it so much, it was about my size). The thick stone walls made it warm and provided great shelter, but it was dark and the ventilation was poor. After an entire winter locked up in here, the animals had exuded a lot of smells. The most pungent and pathological of these was the ammonia from cow urine.

There were about sixty calves in the shed, they'd been born there over the winter and they hadn't seen the outside world, nor breathed the beautiful crisp air just outside the door. I knew what the problem was without looking, but I dutifully examined the ten calves that were sick. I placed the stethoscope on their chests: wheezes, rasps, rattles and rales – a cacophony of bad sounds that just shouldn't have been there. Some also had high temperatures, and two in particular were very sick.

''Tis their lungs, eh lad?'

Mr Evans had his suspicions, but I think my facial expression had given it away. It was a very bad respiratory-tract disease that could kill them unless we turned things around. Mr Evans told me that he changed the flooring every so often, but maybe not as often as he should. This allowed the urine and hence the ammonia to build up, causing the problem. I'd seen this sort of disease in feedlots in Australia. To cure it we were going to have to use very strong antibiotics, but even then I wasn't confident of overcoming the underlying problem.

I turned to Mr Evans. 'You've got sixty calves and these ten are sick. Those fifty over there are about to get sick. We've got to do something about it. Can we get them outside?'

'Ooo, nooo. We can't. They've got to stay in the shed.'

I knew if they stayed in the shed he was facing a disaster. We had to come up with a plan, and eventually we worked one out whereby he let the cows and calves out into a little field next to the shed for most of the day, before bringing them back in at night. That allowed him to clean out the shed more and ensure better hygiene. He had to sacrifice the grass in that field, but the calves thrived. They flourished, and the respiratory-tract disease dissipated with all the clean air.

With Caroline focused on the small animals, John and I did all the on-call work. When the farmers rang you in the middle of the night, they would often start speaking Welsh expecting to get John. It was quite a disorientating thing to hear this strange babble on the other end of the line when you'd just woken up. *Who am I and what am I doing here?*

'Sorry. What? Who? Sorry, I don't speak Welsh.'

'Ooo. Where are you from?' I could tell they were almost daring me to say England so that they could adjust their contempt accordingly.

'I'm from Australia.'

'That's good, then,' and they would continue on in friendly tones. They were very proud of their language, with all its quirks. Double 'l' sounds abounded, vowels seemed in short supply and the words were impossibly long. The older farmers spoke Welsh as their first language, but it had petered out until it was re-embraced a few years ago. My age cohort in Abergele almost all attended Welsh-speaking schools. Northern Wales was a real stronghold of the language; it was less frequently spoken in the south where they also had a different dialect. One farmer, an avid rugby fan, blamed this difference for the national team's poor performances. 'One half of the team has no idea what the other half is saying.'

I learnt most of my Welsh from road signs, which were in Welsh and English, providing a direct translation for me as I drove around lost. I spent a lot of time being lost. Many of the roads don't have names or signposts. John would give me directions like: 'You go along there for 3 miles and you take the second real turning on the left after the church, which is just on the bend. You go up there for a while, then cross the river in the glen and there'll be a sign to a church and you take that for 2 miles and the farm's on the left.'

'Right. Okay.'

So I'd write it all down and leave confidently with these directions. But soon my certainty would evaporate, and I'd be wondering if that was a 'real turning' or an 'unreal turning'. I spent a lot of time completely bamboozled in the Rover. All the lanes were hedged. The hedges acted as fences and windbreaks between fields. The problem was that they also acted as mazes. And there was the constant threat of an oncoming car; the lanes only fitted one vehicle. Thankfully, most of the farmers got around in high-top vans. It rained so much that open utes like we use in Australia were impractical. I could see the Ford Transit vans over the hedges so I could at least get out of the way. The Rover had a lot of bumps and scratches and I added a few more having to ditch it into the hedge when I met another vehicle at speed in the lanes, grinding to a halt with a squeal of brakes, a rustling of the hedge and the dull thud of the front bumper hitting soft earth.

But I loved getting lost. Every day I'd see the rolling hills, so green, with beautiful crumbling dark-stone walls around tiny paddocks. The ocean off to the north moved from blue to black with the weather, and on rare days I saw Mount Snowdon.

I was convinced I was in the prettiest pocket of earth on the planet. And I got to spend so much time soaking it up while looking for the second real turning on the left that I became quite an expert at taking photos of it.

HOLEY COW

Anthony

Jack Roberts was on the phone. 'I've got a cow with a bit of a hole in the side of her,' he said.

'Oh, yeah? A hole?' People tend to exaggerate these problems. 'You mean she's cut herself. Is it bleeding?'

'No, it's not bleeding.'

'Okay so it's not that big a hole?'

'Nah, it's quite big.'

'Okay, let's quantify this. Are we talking a golf ball or a soccer ball?'

'Yeah, no … Maybe a soccer ball. Might be bigger though. Depends how you look at it.'

'Okay, I'm coming out straight away. Make sure you've got the cow in the yards. We don't want to spend half an hour chasing a cow with a hole in it.'

Jack's place was a beautiful stud that ran a big red French breed of cattle called Limousin. It was owned by his brother, a wealthy lawyer from Sydney who called the shots. But Jack did all the work and he kept the place and cattle immaculate. I drove out there, up a quiet country lane, wondering what this guy was talking about. He certainly didn't have a way with words.

I arrived to find Jack waiting for me, nervously pacing about, and I could see the deep red form of the cow waiting in the crush as requested. I went straight over to look and it took a while for my brain to adjust to what my eyes were seeing. This cow's skin had been stripped off from the pin bones, back near the tail, forward to the ribs and down to the bottom of the abdomen, so the hide hung down in a huge triangle, dangling to the ground.

I couldn't comprehend it. The cow stood in the crush like she was in a trance. Swaying slowly, but twitchy. I examined her and noticed that she was overtly sensitive to noise and touch. But at the same time she was quiet and absent – like I'd imagine a drug addict who was out to the world to be. I was sure it was a coping mechanism given to her by nature to deal with pain.

'What on earth happened to her?'

'Oh, well, we were moving the cows from one paddock to the next. We brought them past the tractor which was parked on the bend and she was on the inside of the herd as they rushed past the tractor and she got pushed onto the silage forks. Kebabed her. We had to pull her off.'

Silage forks are like the forks on a forklift truck, only bigger and sharper. They're designed to lift those great big bales of fermented hay that you see sitting in paddocks wrapped in light green plastic. So knowing how long the forks were, I went round to the other side of the cow to see if there was any sign of damage there, and sure enough there were two smaller holes – one right up at the top rear and one further forward at the ribs – where the silage forks had gone right through the body and come out the other side. How those forks hadn't hit something vital in their passage and killed her already was a mystery. But it didn't mean she would survive.

'There's nothing we can do for her,' I said. 'We've got to put her down immediately. We can't manage her with these wounds.'

'We can't put her down,' he said. 'It's not my cow. It's my brother's and he always wants to save them. Surely we can do something.'

'I can't. Even if I could fix the internal wounds, I couldn't stitch the skin back. Once a wound gets to a certain size, the blood supply won't come back. So even if I stitched all that skin back, most of it would die from a lack of blood supply.'

Jack scratched his head and looked at the ground. 'Well I can't give you permission to put her down.'

'But I can't manage this cow's pain. We can't manage her with painkillers for the amount of time it would take to heal. And we don't have those types of painkillers anyway.'

'Well, you have to do something because we can't put her down. I'll try to contact my brother to see what he wants.'

'We need to get hold of him right away; this cow is in all sorts of trouble. We can't save her and we can't alleviate her pain; the only thing to do is to put her out of her misery.'

I gave her an enormous dose of painkiller to try to make her a bit more comfortable, but I knew it would wear off quickly.

The cow was in shock. She was standing but barely conscious – quiet and withdrawn and shaking. You could have pushed her over if you'd wanted. She'd lost a lot of blood and so was cold – the body shuts down at the the periphery. As she stood there unsteadily, she'd occasionally bump against the side of the rail on the bad side, then lurch away in pain and bash into the other side.

Jack was trying his best but he didn't know a lot about cows or pain or many other things. He was just under instructions not to kill things. I could have overridden him but you're not the Stasi. You're a private practice trying to manage a relationship with a client.

'We'll get a bloke to come and shoot her,' Jack suggested. That might have been all right but I wasn't confident it would actually happen. I suspected she might get left for a week 'just to see how she goes'. Jack couldn't see any big problem. As far as he was concerned, if she was still standing she couldn't be that bad: stupid vet couldn't stitch her up. Never mind; we'll just see what happens.

I felt that morally I couldn't leave the farm with the animal still alive. It broke my heart to see the state she was in and I wanted it over as soon as possible. It took a frustratingly long time, but we eventually managed to get Jack's brother on the line and I sent him a picture of the cow to prove my point.

He gave immediate permission to put the cow out of its misery and apologised for his brother's behaviour.

SURGICAL CONDITIONS

Anthony

Bob McWhirter was the guy that you wished was your grandfather. Unfortunately, he was a never-married dairy farmer with no kids. When you visited Bob's farm at the bottom of the escarpment, over a couple of shallow weirs, you smelled it before you saw it. The pungent mix of calf shit, rye grass, silage, milk powder and cow dung. Invariably, Bob would be standing outside his little dairy waiting for you. He only milked eighty cows, like they used to in the days before dairy deregulation. Stuck in the past, he did it the old way. He milked alone, got the cows in alone and lived alone. As a result, the area around the dairy was a pigsty. Mud and crap covered every surface. However, it was always a pleasure to visit Bob. The big smile you got when you arrived, the 'Here's Anthony,' closely followed by the, 'No beautiful students in tow today, mate. What's wrong with you?'

I had been called out this day to check a cow that was 'not right'. Bob stood in front of me beaming. He was a thick-set bloke with wiry ginger hair growing from his head, neck and every orifice. He extended his meaty arms for a handshake, revealing fingers like bodybuilders carrying suitcases, and black skin cancers, ominous but ignored, growing over the exposed bits of his arm.

'I've got a few others for you to take a look at while you're here,' he said, leading me through the slosh in his grey Slazenger trackies pulled up impossibly high over his faded blue flanno.

The crush was set at the back of the dairy and you usually ended up shin-deep in the prior milking's filth. Most dairy farmers wash out their entire yard, but Bob didn't see the need to clean out anything that wasn't in the food-producing area.

Our clinic has been tending that dairy for over forty years, right back to George Bouris, and I'm told that my predecessors had never seen it clean either. Interestingly, we were billeting Japanese students recently and Sidney, my then fiancée, was tripping them around for the true Australian experience. With a great Aussie bloke who always gave you the time of day, and a herd of quiet dairy cows, what better place than Bob's? That night I asked Sid what she thought of the place, expecting the worst. She said it was the cleanest dairy she had ever been to. I couldn't believe it, but Geoff Manning confirmed it when he visited the farm the next day. Over all the years of battling infection on this farm, Geoff had never succeeded in rallying Bob to clean up. Send out a pretty blonde with a group of students, however, and you could cook off the floor.

On this particular day, after pregnancy-testing four cows and dehorning a 'killer' steer I came to the cow in question – a leggy, thin old Friesian. You can generally tell the worth of a dairy cow by the size of her udder and how much body fat she is carrying. A quick glance at this one told me she wasn't worth more than burger money. I took it gently though, knowing Bob was a compassionate soul. I asked him the standard questions: her age; stage of lactation; pregnancy status; prior year's milk production; feed intake. And the answers weren't positive.

This cow would normally not need a vet to prescribe truckacillin – a quick drive to the saleyards.

'She is one of my favourites, mate,' Bob said. 'She's one of the oldest cows on the property. She's the last into the dairy each day so she's a great plug.' The 'plug' is the cow that pushes all the other cows up into the yard and the bails. She will walk all the way up the bail, no matter how many cows are in there, and hold the second last cow fast, allowing the milking clusters to be put on safely. They are a big asset on a dairy farm and most farmers are reluctant to lose them; especially one like Bob who didn't have a worker to help him.

'Okay, mate, let's have a look,' I said.

The old head bail didn't work so Bob had to hold her in place with brute force. Not a problem, but inconvenient all the same as I took her temperature, listened to her heart and chest and checked the integrity of her teeth.

'Everything's normal there,' I said. 'Let's check her abdomen. How long since she last calved Bob?'

'About 150 days.'

'Okay.' This made me think that she might have displaced her fourth stomach – the abomasum – and been carrying that problem around for a while. I listened to her right side, the death-sentence side. If I heard a pinging noise like a tap dripping into a steel bucket, it would indicate that her fourth stomach had moved to the right, become blocked and was filled with gas. On the right, this is usually fatal. Thankfully it was all clear. So I had to check that the abomasum hadn't moved to the left, a serious but less severe problem. At a normal dairy, this involves a simple walk to the other side of the crush. But at Bob's farm the left side of the crush wasn't used very much. Except as a manure heap. Cows are prolific pooers. Most dairies have run-off areas, big drains and ponds to handle the enormous volume of crap. At Bob's place, it had all been stored on the left side of the crush.

I was glad I was wearing my full-size gumboots. I clambered over the top of the race and down the other side. When I tentatively put my foot down, it immediately began to sink. I had to get the other one down quick smart to avoid losing my boot. So that was it, I was stuck. Luckily, I was in the right spot to have a listen to the cow's abdomen. I placed the bell of my trusty Littmann stethoscope against her abdomen and began the familiar routine of flicking the skin around the bell of the instrument. The normal sound is the dull thud of a finger on flesh. Unfortunately this time I heard the high-pitched ping – the sound of abnormal gas stuck in a stomach. *Bugger!* A left displacement of the abomasum.

Lastly, I put my hand inside her rectum, felt down through the uterine wall and touched the calf, and sure enough the little bugger almost bit me. This cow wouldn't be ready to calve for a while, but the calf was alive and healthy, and might be just like its mum – a big asset.

The normal procedure would be to lock the cow in place, give it loads of local anaesthetic and a bit of sedation, cut a big hole in the cow's right flank, pull the stomach back around and suture it in place. But the head bail didn't work and the right side of the crush didn't open. It was just an old piece of train track with lots of metal tubing.

I explained the left abomasum displacement to Bob and it was all a bit new to him. 'I've heard of places having it,' he said, 'but we've never had one diagnosed here before.'

I speculated that that might have been because no one else was foolish enough to climb over into the poo pile to listen. Anyway, Bob's immediate reaction was that the cow was buggered and should be sold. Favourite or not, dairy farmers are good at putting sentimentality aside.

'I dunno,' I said. 'I reckon we can save her.'

The idea of surgery was confronting to Bob and, under the circumstances, confronting to me too. I had done quite a lot of them; however, the procedure was still relatively new and a lot of our farmers were yet to be convinced of its worth. I had adopted the policy of doing the first one on each farm 'at cost' to demonstrate its effectiveness. Convincing Bob was a big challenge as well. He stood to make $500 just selling her for meat; if my operation failed he'd get nothing for her.

'But she's got a calf inside her and if it's a heifer that's a big plus for you,' I said.

'All right,' he said. 'Let's give it a go.'

Bugger! I realised I'd done it again; talked my way into a difficult and problematic surgery. I had no way of fixing this cow into the race, and even if I could, I couldn't access her right side. *How on earth am I going to do this?*

Bob looked on, eager, yet suspicious of my motives.

I decided the only thing for it would be to back the cow into the race, tie her head to the rail with a halter, her body to the rail with a rope and go for it standing knee-deep in shit. Imagine if human surgeons operated in such conditions.

A mate from uni who went on to do medicine after graduating as a vet, told me he was once lectured on the technique for an epidural. He had done heaps on cows himself and was busy educating the med students within earshot. The professor called him out and asked what all of the discussion was about. My mate said simply that epidurals weren't that hard. 'You just lift her tail, wipe the shit off and give the injection.' He was immediately ejected from the class, but it wasn't because he was wrong.

The faeces equation in this case was a little too stacked in death's favour. Not only was the surgery site grossly contaminated, I was stuck in place. Even if I had wanted to move I couldn't. My feet were suctioned into the mud and my surgery site had been pre-determined.

This was coupled with Bob sitting atop the yards, smirking down at me while also bemoaning how much the cow was worth as meat. 'Geoff's never done this, you know.'

What am I doing?

I went through all the preliminary stuff – putting in epidurals, local blocks, shaving the hair, prepping the skin. I was ready to go.

A good surgeon is sure of himself and doesn't hesitate. Quick, bold strokes with the scalpel and an economy of energy are what make a good surgeon. And I was determined to be one. You have to push hard when you cut through all that boot leather. So I pushed hard and I was in with just two cuts: one through the skin and one through the three muscle layers that comprise the cow's flank. The negative pressure whistled in my ears as air flowed in. I was happy with myself. It usually took ages for me to get into the abdomen. I put my hand into the cow, searching around for the misplaced stomach. Over the rope holding her in place, over the rumen, down the other side. I was shoulder deep in her guts with my feet stuck in mud and shit when I heard a groan – like a ghost with bellyache. And down she went.

Of course she fell right in the deepest part of the mud, just in front of my toes. And of course she fell with her new wound deepest in the poo. *She is stuffed. I am stuffed. There is no way out of this. Why me?* The look on Bob's face was unforgettable. To me it said, 'I like you … you little shit, but you have buggered my cow and for that I won't forgive you.' The exasperation washed over me. *Why was I trying these new ideas when I could have just diagnosed a terminal gastro problem and put her on the truck? Why did I try?*

But I *was* trying, and there was no backing out now. Bob went off to get the tractor. He took an eternity with me standing anchored in the manure. He came back with the hiplifters on the front and we managed to get the cow back on her feet to reveal a wound that was covered with faeces and sludge so gross that even the flies were avoiding it.

'Will your hose reach the race?' I asked.

'Yeah, I reckon. I'll go get it. And I'll bring the .22 while I'm over there. That'll save a lot of time.'

I was inclined to agree. Blind Freddy could see that this cow was buggered, but I just couldn't let it go. 'Bob, I think we should keep going with the surgery. What have we got to lose?'

'Nah, don't worry about it,' Bob said. 'It'll take too long and cost me even more.'

'Don't worry about the money, Bob. This one's on the house.'

I hosed out the wound and got my arms in and pulled the abomasum through and around. The cow stayed on her feet and everything seemed to go smoothly after that. I marinated that cow in penicillin: some in the abdomen before I stitched up the muscles; some in the muscles before I stitched up the hide; some in the wound. As I extricated my boots from their holes in the slop, I left Bob with strict instructions to give her twice daily injections for a week.

'Yeah, I'll try but I doubt she'll be around that long,' he said.

'You're probably right, but we've come this far. We might as well see.'

The usually exuberant farewells from the grandpa I wished I had were fairly quiet that afternoon. Bob seemed pretty keen to be somewhere else, somewhere sensible. Me too. I left with my tail between my legs.

I avoided the inevitable follow-up call for as long as I could. I just didn't want to hear the bad news for which I would be entirely responsible. However, my love for Bob was too great. I just had to know how he was going and how long the cow had survived before the infection claimed her. Instead of picking up the phone, though, I decided to drop by one afternoon. Bob was obviously surprised to see me, but he was his usual happy self.

I ditched the pleasantries and got straight to the point. 'How's the cow?'

'Great, mate. Last into the dairy as usual and her milk production has come right back up. She is a keeper, well done.' The slap on the back couldn't have felt sweeter. 'I can't understand why we haven't done that operation more often.'

'Yeah, me neither,' I said.

We now do Bob's surgeries at his neighbour's new yards.

BREAKFAST FAR FROM TIFFANY'S

James

The phone rang in the middle of one of my first nights on call.

'It's Mr Jones Ty Coch. Sorry to wake you. I've got a calving. Can you come out?'

'Yeah, sure. Where are you?'

'I'm the Mr Jones at Ty Coch, the farm on the hill near Betws-Yn-Rhos.'

My first problem was that there are only four names in Wales: Jones, Davis, Williams and Evans. And every second farmer with one of those four names lived on a farm called Ty Coch. At least he'd narrowed the field down. There would have only been half a dozen Jones Ty Cochs on a hill near Betws-Yn-Rhos.

'So can you give me directions?'

'Where are you from?' he asked suspiciously.

'Australia.'

I heard him relax. 'Oookay, you go up the hill towards Llanfair and it's on the left. So you go up there and you take the old road that takes you right to Llangernyw. When you reach the power station you take the real left turning there and go along for 3 miles, past the church on the right and then you will take a turning that will take you over the brook and up the other side of the glen and my farm is on the bryn to the right. That's Mr Jones Ty Coch.'

It was 4 a.m. I shivered out of bed, trying to write down the directions. *How am I ever going to find this place?* I drove out into the moonless night. A light mist hung in the air as I negotiated mazes around power stations and unseen brooks, churches and valleys. Being dark, I couldn't even enjoy the scenery.

Somehow I got there about 4.30 a.m. and Mr Jones, short and portly under a tweed cloth cap, walked out into the Rover's single headlight beam to meet me. He shook my hand with his enormous rough paw and showed me to the barn where he had the cow called Bessy tied to a post. Most Australian cows would be having conniptions at such a restraint but British cows are used to being held like this. I put my hand in and tried for some time to sort out the calf inside her but it just wasn't going to come. This cow needed a caesarean. No problems. Mr Jones was used to this. His cattle were of a thick-set European breed that often needed surgical intervention.

'Do you have a crush?' I asked.

'No.'

'Nothing at all like that?'

'No.'

'Where does John do this sort of thing when he comes here?'

'We just tie them up right here.'

'Okay Mr Jones, if it's good enough for John. Let's sort it out.'

It was something I was to learn – that no one seemed to have good sturdy yards with crushes designed to handle boisterous cattle. If you were lucky, you might get half a race with a wiry gate that didn't close properly, or you'd get Mr Jones Ty Coch's set-up which was a post and a halter. So with Bessy attached to the post, Mr Jones tied an extra loop around her belly to secure her to the wall of the barn. She was somewhat immobilised but if we upset her she'd easily break free. I put in the anaesthetic, prepped her up and cut into her. All the while, there was a peanut gallery of cows watching from a higher slope. The barn was the size of two tennis courts. It was divided into different areas and all the cows were lined up along the dividers watching in total silence in the pre-dawn stillness. No birds sang outside. There was just me and Mr Jones, Bessy and her silent friends.

The operation went well. Bessy stood there passively while I pulled a large live bull calf from her abdomen, which always brought a small sense of wonder, no matter how many times I delivered one. But that sense was about to be magnified ten-fold as I stitched Bessy up and looked over her back to see daylight starting to filter through ventilation gaps in the wall behind her. I'd arrived in darkness so had no idea where I was. But as the beautiful soft light started to wash over us, I realised that I was in fact on a wondrously beautiful hillside looking out across the Irish Sea. The creeping daylight revealed hedges and hills bisected by tumbledown stone fences. I absorbed all this over the top of the cow on which I'd just performed a successful operation in not-so-ideal conditions. It was absolutely glorious. Magical. And I didn't need any reminders about why I loved this job and why I was here.

Mr Jones Ty Coch lived with this splendour every day. For him it was just another morning, except with the inconvenience and cost of having the vet out.

I was trying to clean up all my gear and squeeze it into the back of the Rover when Mr Jones called out to his wife in Welsh. The farmers would often slip back into their native tongue. She called something unintelligible back and then he turned to me. 'You'll be joining us for breakfast.'

I wasn't sure if it was a question or a command. 'What … um. Yes. Yes.'

'My wife is cooking it now.'

So I finished the packing and hosed myself off. It was viciously cold despite the beautiful sunrise as I made my way across to the ancient whitewashed cottage with its tiny windows and amazing view.

Mrs Jones, a rosy-cheeked, friendly woman of about sixty, soon presented a marvellous spread of bacon, eggs and black pudding with beautiful home-baked bread. It was getting towards 7 a.m. I was meant to be back at work so I ate quickly to assuage the guilt.

'You've got to have another cup of tea, lad,' Mrs Jones said.

'I've got to get going. I don't want to be late for John.'

'John! Don't you worry about John. He always has breakfast when he comes here and he takes hours. He's always saying I can squeeze in one more before Caroline will miss me.'

I had the extra cup with a slice of thickly buttered bread before returning to the Rover. In the short time I'd been driving it, I'd grown to hate this car. It was really just a rebadged Honda Civic, and it was amazing that in the simple act of changing its name they'd turned it into a junkyard dog of a car. It was faded maroon, had only one hubcap, the radio didn't work, and it made a whirring noise when driving like it was being powered by propellers. I never knew which gear I was in, but generally if the gearstick was in my crotch I was probably in fifth. And with no compartment to separate dirty clothes and equipment from the driver's cabin, it smelt like a dairy floor. Worst of all it broke down a lot. So every time I got into the Rover it was with a small sense of dread. But this day it sped me back to work like a Jaguar and I trotted in with my full belly and a rich sense of satisfaction.

I told John and Caroline I'd been called out to a calving.

'That's fine,' John said. 'Where did you go?'

'Had to go out to Mr Jones Ty Coch.'

'Oh yes. Which Mr Jones Ty Coch?' John asked.

We would have this problem all the time. For billing purposes, there were so many farmers with the same names I'd have to explain to

John what he looked like, or if he spoke Welsh or English, or what his jokes were like, for John to deduce which of the Jones Ty Cochs I was talking about.

I told him about the little white cottage and the stunning ocean view.

'Oh yes, I know the one. Did you get breakfast?'

'Yes, I did, as a matter of fact.'

'Is that why you're late?'

'It was a very nice meal, thank you very much. I ate it quickly though. I tried to escape as soon as I could but they said you always stayed for breakfast.'

'Yes, they're very gracious hosts.'

Just then, Caroline, who had been off elsewhere, re-entered the conversation. 'Who's a gracious host?' she asked.

I began to explain: 'After I'd done the caesarean, I –'

'He couldn't get the damned Rover started,' John interrupted. 'Mr Jones helped him get it going again. A very gracious old chap. Must get that thing serviced.'

DOUBLE TROUBLE

Anthony

The red-and-white Poll Hereford cow frothed at the mouth. Her bulging eyes were fixed on us as she attempted to jump the high metal rails that enclosed her. She couldn't make the height, and her legs tangled with the railings as she fell back. Flailing on the ground only momentarily, she rushed straight back to her feet to bellow and stare and snort at us before mounting another attack. She didn't want to escape the yards. She wanted to hurt us.

I'd only just got out of my car. A local shop owner named James Chatfield had rung me less than an hour earlier: 'I've got a cow trying to calve but something's wrong. I don't have time to do it myself, so can you come and have a look? She's a real nice quiet cow so she won't give you any strife. Her name's Maree. She's the family pet.'

It was a sticky, hot February day. Aside from this family pet's apparent mood swing, the first thing I noticed about her was the stench. This cow stank of death and she was being followed by a cloud of flies. If every fly on the South Coast wasn't there, they mustn't have got the memo. I thought it was probably septic shock. The calf had presumably died inside her and now the toxins from the putrefaction were playing havoc with her brain.

James's father-in-law, Bill, was there to help and our first task was to get this cow into the crush so we could get a look at her. We opened the required gates and I stood on top of the rails – on the outside – and waved my arms trying to look tall. She saw me and charged. I jumped back as she crashed into the fence. She spun around and ran at a gate, preparing to leap. Her body lifted and for a moment it looked like she was going to get over the 6-foot-high metal barrier, but her legs tangled on the rails and she hung there momentarily before falling onto her back. If she'd got out, she would've been gone. No barbed-wire fence could have held her snorting fury. She might not have hated me personally but she very clearly wanted me gone.

You don't herd these animals anywhere. You just open the gates you want them to go through and give them the merest suggestion of the direction they should go in. Then you stand back and hope. Eventually her crazy rampage took her down the race and we were able to catch her neck in the head crush. She thrashed around a bit, but she soon calmed down with the restraint. I donned a shoulder-length glove and swung the half-gate around that stopped her kicking backwards and went in to investigate. Sure enough, there was a calf inside her in the breech position; it had been coming for a long time and was rotten, rotten, rotten. Generally when you do a rotten calving, the flesh of the calf is decomposed to the texture of, say, cooked chicken. You pull on the flesh and it tears apart, like slow-cooked meat. It's been in the oven at 37 degrees for three weeks, after all. But this calf had been there for so long even the bones had gone soft.

A caesarean wasn't an option because when they're this rotten the uterus itself is starting to decay so as soon as you put a knife in it collapses and releases all the muck. Just the simple act of operating on this animal would likely kill it. Luckily I didn't need to do a caesarean because the cervix, while not fully open, was wide enough for me to get two hands through. So I got cracking. It was stinking hot and I was wearing overalls, but at least I had the shade of a tree above. Bill was good for conversation but not a cow man. We chatted away about the cricket and the weather as I pulled the calf out one mushy piece at a time. Pretty soon my gloves had been shredded by the shards of bone.

I got the back legs out okay, then got to work on the rib cage. Because it was coming out backwards, however, the ribs were facing the wrong way so they caught like barbs along the birth canal. I had to break every rib and pull them out one by one. It took a lot of strength doing it with my arm fully outstretched, just using the leverage from the wrist. I absorbed heat from the cow and the sun, and was sweating like I'd dipped my head in a bucket. I desperately wanted to wipe my brow and swat the flies away from my eyeballs but I couldn't because of the fetid juices on my hands. I tried to keep up a pleasant banter with Bill but it was so hard.

What am I doing? Why am I a vet? There are easier ways to make a living. Why didn't James call me weeks ago? How did he not know something was wrong?

I knew that James hadn't known anything was wrong. I continued with the job and got on to breaking the spine because it wouldn't come out either. I also snapped the shoulder blades. I got the front legs out all right, but the cervix had started to shrink even in the time I'd been there, and the head wouldn't come. Still inside the uterus, I had to cut the head in half with gili wire.

After a bit of a wrestle, I got the last piece of skull out and tossed it onto the pile of soggy hair, putrid bones, flesh and skin just behind me. After an hour and half of the worst job I'd ever done, I managed a joke with Bill. 'Hope it's not twins.'

'Don't say that,' he said. 'You'll regret it.'

I wasn't worried. The calf was too big to be a twin. But any good vet will always put their hand back in at the end to check for spares and tears in the uterus. I was exhausted, but I inserted my hand, fished around for a bit, then called back to Bill. 'How many legs can you count on the ground?'

He got up and had a poke through the 2-foot-high and 4-foot-wide pile of rot.

'Four,' he said.

I had a fifth leg in my hands. 'Far out! It's twins.'

It was like reaching the top of a mountain only to see that the real peak was hundreds of metres above. My hands were cut and bruised, the muscles were stuffed. I had unspeakable gunk packed so far under my nails it felt like they were going to fall off. And I had to repeat the whole process.

The second calf was smaller and facing in the correct direction but I still had to break bits of it off to bring it through the shrinking cervix. I finally got it out and gave the cow an enormous dose of penicillin – five times the standard dose. I gave her anti-inflammatory painkillers to reduce the pain and hold the shock in check. But there was still a major problem.

You can't imagine the cesspool of putrid garbage that was still inside Maree's uterus. The amniotic fluid was now a soup of fur and blood and puss and guts. It seemed hopeless. *How can this cow survive?* She was already septic. I couldn't scoop this stuff out.

So I said to Bill, 'Can you go and get a garden hose that reaches here and turn it on?'

He got me a new green hose. I took off the nozzle and stuck it inside the cow, just letting the water run into the uterus. It took a while for Maree to fill up but eventually all the gunk started pouring out the birth canal. I let it run until the water went clear. It cleaned her out and cooled her down.

Sure I was exhausted, I was covered from head to toe in putrescent muck and 300 bazillion flies, but there was that sense of achievement. I'd set out to do this job. I'd done it and given the cow the best possible chance of surviving.

Yes, this is why I'm a vet.

'Okay I think we're done. Let's let her go.'

We opened the head bail and stepped well clear. The craziness that had possessed Maree seemed to have been exorcised. She wobbled out, tentative and unsteady, like you'd expect after such an ordeal, but calm. She turned and looked at me with an air of serenity, and for the first time I could see the lovely family pet that she was. Then she knelt shakily down on her front legs, followed by her back legs, bringing her belly to rest on the ground. She gave a huge sigh and went still.

Worried, I snuck into the field and crept up behind her, because I still wasn't certain all her demons had departed. As I approached, I saw no sign of movement, no breathing, and once I plucked up the courage to kneel down beside her, I felt no heartbeat.

I lost it. I did my lolly. I screamed and yelled and kicked things and determined that there obviously was no God, but I was so tired my kicks were pretty limp – they barely knocked the bucket over. And my curses were fairly lame.

Bill just stayed a safe distance from me. I think he thought I looked a bit like that cow prior to getting her into the crush. Eventually he herded me back towards the car, maybe opened the door and turned on the air-con, giving me the merest suggestion of the direction he wanted me to go, and quietly backed away.

RESPIRATORY RODENTS

James

John and Caroline had a branch practice five minutes down the A55 at Deganwy, a beautiful harbour town with a castle on the hill. I'd been there a week and was settling in nicely thanks to the nurse, Olive, who was a friendly giant; tall with big curly black hair that looked just a little out of control. When she spoke she had the same soothing tone as the nurses when I was a kid telling me that everything was going to be fine.

I was working my way through the morning consults, feeling hungry and very keen to get back to the excellent sandwich shop next door when Olive walked in. 'Mrs Williams has got a wee patient for you. Some skin issues.'

Mrs Williams was standing in the waiting room and holding a tiny box, about 20 by 20 centimetres, covered with a towel.

Mmmmm, very small container. Wonder what it is?

'Noticed some skin problems have we, Mrs Williams?' I said in my jolly and confident medical voice.

'Yes, he's got a little bit of a rash and I think he might be a little raspy in his chest,' she said.

'Okay, I'll have a little look and we'll see what we find.'

She took the towel off to reveal a small orange cage. It was all I could do not to scream out, 'Holy rat poo! What is that?' I'd never seen such a creature before. It was some type of rodent, but tiny; maybe 3 centimetres high and 4 centimetres long, with big ears and a little tail.

'Yes, yes,' I said. Unable to think of anything else to say, I channelled my inner Ben and repeated myself. 'Yes, yes.'

A golden rule of veterinary science is that when you don't have the foggiest idea of what you're doing, you reach for the stethoscope. I grabbed mine, hanging at my chest, and the creature pretty much disappeared as I put the metal disc to its body. I listened to its crazily fast heartbeat and nodded knowingly. 'Yes, yes. Okay. This stethoscope is a little big. I might see if I've got a smaller one.'

I excused myself from the consult room. The clinic was tiny and the paper-thin walls did not go all the way to the ceiling. So you could hear everything that was going on in the whole clinic. I could just about hear my diminutive patient breathing from the reception area. Olive was there doing some paperwork and I stood behind her waving like I was drowning.

Fortunately she did not offer to give mouth to mouth but instead made a 'What's wrong?' face.

I made a scribbling motion with my hand and she handed me a pen and paper. I wrote, 'What is that?' and she looked at me with an uncomprehending tilt of the head.

I drew an arrow to the consult room, and wrote, 'What is that animal?'

She took the pad and pen off me and wrote, 'Hamster.'

I realised that I'd never actually seen a hamster before. I furrowed my brow, screwed up my nose and whispered. 'Aren't hamsters guinea pig-sized?'

'No. That's a hamster, dear.'

'Okay, yes. Yes ... good ... yes, yes.'

Hamsters are illegal in Australia because of the risk of them going feral so they were not something that we were taught about extensively (read: at all) at university. I had to go and find the *Manual of Exotic Pets*, a book put out by the British Small Animal Veterinary Association. It was very straightforward, using simple language as though it was written specifically for young Australian vets who hadn't the foggiest.

'Just looking for that stethoscope, Mrs Williams,' I called out while furiously scanning the index and flicking the pages. 'Olive tells me there's a small one here somewhere.'

I read the hamster passage quickly. The book was gold. I made a presumptive diagnosis of a bacterial infection both of the skin and the respiratory tract. It seemed relatively early in the course of the disease so hopefully we could get him back on track, but it indicated that there were some imbalances in his body. As I quickly read up about it I found that hamsters have a lifespan of about two years. Now, when I asked Mrs Williams how old hers was I could figure out whether it was young, old or middle aged.

I walked back in with a newfound confidence and a stethoscope that looked remarkably like the previous one. I listened to its pulse again. 'Oh yes, that's much clearer now. Yes, yes. I think he's got an imbalance of the bacteria in the body, and it's allowing the infection of the respiratory tract and the skin. It's a relatively common condition and you've got to it fairly early, Mrs Williams, so hopefully he'll respond to the therapy. We'll need to treat him with antibiotics and we'll expect him to get better in the next week, but we're going to have to manage it going forward.'

Mrs Williams was clearly impressed by my deep knowledge of hamster biology and pathology. The hamster got better and she probably thinks to this day that I knew what I was talking about. Indeed, I did my research and learnt that Mrs Williams had a dwarf Russian hamster. Who knew that there was more than one type? I locked that away in my head for future use and even now I always have a copy of the *Manual of Exotic Pets* at hand.

Abergele was a much more intensive small-animal practice than I'd worked in before. We did a lot of complex medical management of cases. We treated diabetic and Cushingoid animals – those with an excess of cortisone in the body – and feline hyperthyroidism, in which older cats get a hormonal imbalance that leads to a ravenous appetite at the same time as weight loss. In Barraba, people had been reticent to treat and investigate these diseases, but in Britain we diagnosed them far more frequently. And the clients seemed far more determined to treat them as actively as possible. Even those from lower socio-economic groups seemed resolute in doing the very best for their pets.

Suddenly, amid all these animal-loving Brits, my vow to the Royal College of Veterinary Surgeons to place the welfare of animals above that of humans didn't seem so odd. It wasn't long before I had to face a case where I had to put the animal's well-being above my own in order to treat it.

A few weeks after the hamster incident, someone brought in another coughing rodent. Except this one was enormous, with a furry tail and great flapping ears.

Fortunately, Olive was more au fait with my ignorance this time and let me know that it was a chinchilla.

A chinchilla? Isn't that a town in Queensland?

I picked the rodent up to have a look and was immediately struck by how it had the most gorgeously soft fur I'd ever encountered. I would have stood there and luxuriated in its velvety silkiness, perhaps nestling it against my cheek, if it wasn't for the fact that I could feel my eyes starting to bulge.

My rabbit allergy had continued since childhood so I avoided those creatures as much as possible, but it was difficult as a vet, especially in the UK where there are so many pet rabbits. If I was at the Deganwy clinic where I was the only vet, rabbit avoidance was doubly difficult. But now I had found a new pointy-nosed foe. I realised I was also allergic to chinchillas. I set this one down and went out the back to pop some antihistamines. I came back to have another quick look and I realised the antihistamines weren't enough. I felt my lungs constricting. I rushed out the back again to inhale feverishly on my Ventolin while I read the *Manual of Exotic Pets*. The client could hear me puffing away on the sprayer, sneezing and snotting as I read that the chinchilla was a rodent native to the high Andes, that it lived in groups called 'herds', and not surprisingly it was in danger of overhunting by the fur industry.

I arrived at a diagnosis of enteritis and prescribed it some antibiotics, telling the owner (a Mrs Jones/Williams/Evans/Davis) that the chinchilla should improve quickly, and to return tomorrow, preferably when John was there, if it didn't.

I came back in and Olive noticed my red eyes and sneezing and the profuse discharge from my nose.

'Are you allergic to these?' she asked.

'Judging by what's going on, I don't think the chinchilla and I are going to be friends.'

The chinchilla's fur is much finer than a rabbit's, so my reaction was much more severe. After the consult I had to take myself off to the doctor who gave me some injections to calm my immune system down.

It remains the only chinchilla I've ever seen, but I will never, ever forget how wonderfully soft that fur was.

NIPPLE CRIPPLE

Anthony

'Who are you? Are you a vet?' someone yelled down the phone.

'Ye ...'

'I don't know. I'm new here. Rebecca's got a tick. I can't get it off and now she won't let me near her.'

You can tell a lot about a person by the way they get you out of bed in the middle of the night. When reasonable people call you in the wee hours, they have usually put the call off until it is absolutely necessary. When they do finally phone, they are extremely apologetic for disturbing your sleep. It's known as common courtesy. And we are only too happy to do everything we can to help them.

'I'm sorry. Who is this?' I asked, maintaining my best professional tone.

'It's a paralysis tick,' the female voice shrieked. 'It'll kill her if we can't get it out. I know this, I've been studying it on the internet. Now Rebecca won't let me go near her. We can't get it out. What can we do?'

'Well, you should ...'

'Google says we should put metho on it but we can't. Rebecca has run into the corner and she's trying to bite us. What are the symptoms

202

of paralysis tick? Does it make them go psychotic? Rebecca has turned psychotic.'

You're not kidding, I thought. *You know what they say about pets resembling their owners.*

'She's a beautiful dog normally. I read on the internet ...'

It was like the three apostles. Woken up in the middle of the night, a rude client and now Dr Google. She was a broken fire hydrant of words just gushing out. I tried to sneak out of bed, but this woman's voice was so loud it was waking my partner. It was almost waking the neighbours. It's bad enough for the partner to be woken by the phone ringing but she could have slipped back to sleep if there wasn't so much commotion.

In the darkness of my home I allowed myself a few eye rolls and the odd grimace as I held the phone out at half an arm's length from my ear, wondering when it might be that I could return to the comfort of bed, but knowing that sleep was now unlikely.

I gathered I was dealing with a couple who were newly moved to the area from Sydney. I suspected they had no children. Rebecca was obviously their proxy child. They'd heard about paralysis ticks and were worried. We worry about paralysis ticks too. If someone finds a paralysis tick on their dog in the middle of the night, we tell them to bring the dog straight in. Even if an animal appears fine, it can go downhill quickly, and the best treatment is early attention.

Eventually the deluge of words subsided enough for me to get in a few questions.

'Now, what's your name?'

'Miriam.'

'Where on Rebecca's body is the tick?'

'On her belly.'

'What colour is it?'

'Black.'

'Okay … um, look, paralysis ticks are white or light blue. If it's black, it's unlikely to be paralysis tick.'

'No, I'm sure it's a paralysis tick. How do you know it's not?'

Because I'm the vet, I thought. 'Because of the colour.' I said.

I tried to explain but she wouldn't believe me. There was no way I was going to talk her out of her diagnosis and her plan of treatment: that Rebecca needed to be in intensive care immediately.

'It's up to you. I'll come in and see you at the clinic, but it'll cost you over $100.'

'That's fine. We're coming.'

So over they came from Kangaroo Valley. It's only a 25-minute drive, but it's a difficult one; climbing 400 metres in altitude up over Berry Mountain, dodging wombats and negotiating steep hairpins, then repeating the process to descend 400 metres to Berry on the coastal plain. I was living a few hundred metres from the clinic, so I just had to stroll over and open the door.

Miriam and her husband, Ben, came bustling through the door exactly twenty-five minutes after I'd put the phone down. Stick-thin with a dark fading beauty, Miriam wore black tights and a cashmere jumper. Ben looked every bit the retired banker in corduroy and thick white woollen pullover.

Rebecca was a Chinese shar-pei, an animal bred as guard dogs with a face so ugly it could scare intruders away. Tolerating strangers was not part of the shar-pei's make-up. Rebecca behaved just fine at first. Until Miriam put her on the table for me to look at.

Rebecca snapped and growled and contorted the fleshy rolls of skin on her face to convince me that no way was I going anywhere near her torso. Fortunately, I didn't have to. It took only a few seconds to diagnose the problem.

'That's a nipple,' I said. 'You've been trying to remove Rebecca's nipple.' I motioned them to the door, unsure if I should laugh or shout at them. 'I'll see you later.'

'No, that's not right,' Miriam said. 'Don't you think I know what a nipple looks like?'

'You see the one you've been trying to pull off? The one the dog will no longer allow you and your long fingernails anywhere near? Well, here, see the other nine identical ticks all lined up in nice symmetrical rows? They're nipples.'

Miriam would not, could not, suffer this. She was convinced the dog was psychotic. Maybe the mental state was being caused by toxins from a cancer, she said.

I continued trying to convince her but then started to lose my cool. 'If I tried to pull your nipple off I'm pretty sure you wouldn't let me near you either.'

'What if it *is* cancer?' Miriam said.

'I don't think it's cancer. I know it's the dog's nipple.'

'How can you be sure it's not cancer?'

'Okay, the way we can be sure is that you bring the dog back tomorrow. I'll surgically remove the remainder of the nipple. We'll take chest X-rays and ultrasounds and full blood tests and it'll cost you about $1000.'

'That sounds good. I'll see you when the clinic opens,' she said.

At last I was able to usher them out the door and lock up. I had at least given them a small face-saving option. Of course they wouldn't get the tests done. In the clarity of daylight they would realise their error and we'd all be left in peace. Sleep, however, was a distant memory for me that night. My exasperation had fired me up as much as if Miriam had come after *my* nipples instead. I tossed and turned, waiting for the first sign of light so I could get up.

I turned up for work with a fog in my head like the clouds that linger up on Berry Mountain. But it all cleared spot on 9 a.m. when

Miriam came through the door demanding action. 'We're ready for that cancer test,' she screeched, standing in the middle of the waiting room. 'If it *is* cancer, she's not going to die, is she? Perhaps I should take her back to Sydney. Our vet there would know what to do. He has much more experience than you. How many dogs have you treated with cancer? You don't look old enough to be a vet. Are you going to do the X-rays here or not? I don't want Rebecca taken anywhere else for X-rays. I don't know what I'd do if she died.'

For her part, Rebecca had bounded in like they were having a fine old adventure. Any resentments from her nightmarish nipple cripple the night before had long since vanished. But Miriam insisted we subject the poor dog to the full palaver of tests.

The pathologist's report came back the next Friday saying that the tissue sample we had taken was in keeping with an inflamed nipple. I rang Miriam to give her the good news. She received it with no hint of an admission that she might have been a tad over-concerned. I couldn't hold my tongue. 'Next time you try to remove your dog's nipple, could you do it on Mondays or Wednesdays when Geoff is on call? He's very experienced. He'll know what to do.'

DAINTY HANDS MAKE LIGHT WORK

James

James Herriot wrote that for ten months of the year sheep are just white dots on green hillsides, but for the other two months they fill the vet's life with work and wonder and disappointment as the lambs start to come. That isn't true for Australian vets. To us, sheep are more like off-white dots on brown hillsides for the entire year. Despite there being tens of thousands of sheep around Barraba and Manilla, I rarely saw one in a veterinary capacity. It's not financially viable for a farmer to call a vet for an animal that is worth about the same as the call-out fee.

When I arrived at Abergele and John was showing me around, he took me out the back to a shed with a washing machine and other bits and pieces in it. Among them was a strange stainless-steel table with a half-crescent bend and railings down both sides.

'What on earth is this?' I'd asked, knowing that it must have some veterinary function.

'It's a sheep caesarean trolley.'

'What?'

John must have picked up my expression of ignorance. 'What happens,' he explained, 'is that when they're lambing and they have trouble, the farmer puts the sheep in their van and brings 'em in. If we can't get them out, we do a caesarean on this table.'

In my two years in Barraba I'd only done one sheep caesarean – on a prized dorper ewe. From my limited experience (did I mention that I won the HC Belschner Prize in Sheep and Wool at uni?) I knew sheep caesareans didn't take long. Twenty-five minutes if you were quick.

'Right, and what do we charge for this?'

'About forty quid.'

And so it was that as the earth started to warm through March and April – so that instead of being miserably cold it was just darned cold – the grass started to grow, the ground dried and the hillsides filled with white dots unleashed from the sheds. Among them were even smaller dots, the lambs experiencing the joy of frolicking and gambolling on grass so green that it was hard to look at. And along with the new lambs arriving, the sheep caesarean trolley became more than just another piece of gear cluttering the shed. The phone would ring in the middle of the night. It would be a crusty farmer slipping between English and Welsh waking me from my beautiful slumber, and once he'd ascertained I wasn't English he'd tell me he was coming in with a ewe. I'd wander downstairs, pull my overalls over my pyjamas and wait for the van to pull up. He'd bring the sheep in, usually a Welsh breed called a Lleyn, often crossed with a Texel or Dorset breed. The Welsh farmers struggled to perform lambings that involved reaching inside the sheep. To a man, they had these enormous hands. No matter how small their stature, hanging on the end of their arms were huge fleshy paddles. I had the advantage of possessing dainty hands which were very useful for manipulating limbs inside a sheep.

'Oh, laddy, if I had hands like that, lambing would be a breeze,' they'd tell me.

John was very happy to have me on board because he had Welsh farmer hands too. But, little hands or not, sometimes I just couldn't get the lambs out. Often it would be twins or triplets all tangled up inside.

There's a very limited space within a ewe to get in and manipulate things around, so you often proceed to the caesarean.

Sheep are fascinating. They run away from you, but if you catch a sheep and tip it over onto its bum, it doesn't fight. It just gives up. They're like: 'Hey, I'm a prey animal. I've achieved my destiny. Come and eat me.'

So we'd lay a sheep on the table with the farmer holding her head. We'd tie the legs and then loop the rope under the table and back over the sheep just in front of the back legs, then do the same across the front. I might sometimes sedate the sheep but usually not. We'd put a local in for pain but they wouldn't need sedation. They'd just patiently wait to be eaten. I'd shave up the side, quickly prep it up, make my incision, go in and within minutes I'd be pulling out twins or triplets all knotted together. I'd stitch up the uterus, then the muscle, hand the farmer the lamb and the ewe, unzip my overalls and go back to bed.

Sometimes, however, I'd look out and there'd be another two vans outside waiting. The number would vary between none and four in a single night on-call. It was an amazing process that just does not happen in Australia.

I asked John why he charged so little for it.

'Well sheep are worth about £100,' he said. 'If we charged any more, they wouldn't come. We don't make any money out of the operation but we provide it as a service. That way the farmers can justify having them and coming to us for their other problems.'

It made sense and was a good lesson in community service. Lambing was also good fun and I can say I've done more sheep caesareans than most Aussie vets – all within a two-month window of my career. After that window closed, sheep went back to being mere white dots on green hills with even smaller dots chasing them around. The caesarean trolley went back to cluttering the shed – unless we were using it as a very fast way down the hill to the George and Dragon … but that's another story.

A GOOD JUDGE OF CHARACTER

Anthony

You get screamed down by the behaviourists if you start to say that dogs hate you. That is anthropomorphic, they'll say. You're giving human traits to animals. The current wisdom is that animals remember you, but it's not hate they are expressing with their low growls and flashing teeth. It's fear. In the same way, it is said that animals don't defend people. People like to tell stories about how, when they were attacked, the dog jumped in to protect them, but apparently it's not true. The dog responds out of fear.

As a vet, you see a lot of animals and the majority are indifferent until you stick something in them. Sometimes, however, one will instantly despise you for no good reason, while others will take an immediate liking to you. When a client brings in an animal that takes a shine to you, you puff up your chest and tell the client their animal is a good judge of character. When they hate you, you scratch your head and comment that there's no good reason for this.

Which brings me to the story of Carol and her dogs. We'd come to call our Tuesday rounds to Shoalhaven Heads 'the widow run'. At the time, the Heads was a quiet little seaside town of mismatched houses and tranquil waters. Retired couples would move down from Sydney to the lovely holiday destination they'd enjoyed throughout their working lives. They sold in Sydney, bought in the Heads and used the leftover to live on. But the husbands had a tendency to die first, leaving the wives stuck there with the family pet, financially unable to return to Sydney. I'd go around and visit them – they really liked the company and I loved it too, getting out on the road in my Magna.

I remember the heavy smoker Edna Meadows coughing in unison with her dog, whose fluffy coat had discoloured like a smoker's moustache. The dog had emphysema. Edna had it too. There is good evidence to suggest that pets that live in smoking households have a much higher incidence of primary lung tumours. Passive smoking pets. Edna's house was always full of smoke and each time I left I'd be coughing along with her and the dog. One time Edna locked herself out and I had to boost her up and through an open window. It was awkward, hoisting this 80-year-old woman with her skirt dangling over my head, but I saw it as part of the community service that we offered. I really did feel that my role out there was greater than just looking after animals.

There was another client, Carol Doulman, who took an instant liking to me, and me to her. She had a mousy-tan silky terrier cross called Bubbles, which was all over me from the very first time I walked in the door. Carol thought I was the bee's knees because the dog loved me, and he was clearly a good judge of character, she said, as he licked my face while I tried to get my nose away from his chronic bad breath. I should have corrected her on the character thing because it was to come back to haunt me.

Despite Bubbles' apparent energy on that very first visit, Carol said the dog was down and flat. When I managed to hold him still long enough to get the stethoscope to his chest I heard the whooshing of turbulent blood flow, like the sound of a skier sloshing down the hill, instead of the crisp 'lub dub, lub dub' that you want to hear. I diagnosed a heart valve insufficiency and later confirmed it with an ultrasound. Basically the heart valves wouldn't shut properly. It is the most common heart disease in small dogs.

We managed Bubbles pretty intensively with diuretics and drugs to increase the efficiency of his heart. I told Carol we weren't fixing the problem, we were just masking it, but Bubbles responded well and bounced back with all his old energy, so she was pretty happy. I was seeing a lot of her, prescribing and delivering medications. I'd always try to leave her visit until the end of my run because then I could linger for a cuppa and chat without leaving other clients waiting. Carol was about seventy-five, slim, with short brown hair and the eyes of someone who'd lived through tough times. She'd travelled a lot, following her husband around the outback with his work, and she exuded that bush spirit of resourcefulness and bluntness. She reminded me of my grandmother.

It got to the point where I'd stop by Carol's house on my Tuesday run whether I needed to see Bubbles or not. We'd have tea and a biscuit and we'd chat at her kitchen table with its green vinyl top tacked down to the wood. I told her about my background and she told me all about her husband and kids and the difficulties of raising a family that was constantly moving. She told me of how, when she lived in the Northern Territory, the tank water got so hot that you could only shower at night. Even then it was almost scalding. It was a world away and I loved her stories.

Sometimes I dropped in on my day off. When I sold the Magna and bought a ten-year-old Subaru WRX that was insanely fast and obnoxiously loud, I picked her up and took her for a drive one afternoon. She was keen for the outing but when I showed her what the car could do I think she regretted coming.

Not long after our drive, Carol rang. As soon as she said hello I knew it wasn't good. 'Anthony, he's dying.'

I'd told her to expect this progression of the disease. The drugs can keep them good for a few years but eventually they crash. She knew what was coming. I drove straight there and found Bubbles barely able to lift his head. I took him back to the clinic on a towel in the back of the car and over the next couple of days gave him fluids and intravenous medication … but try as we did, I think we all knew it was hopeless.

And so, with great sadness, I put Bubbles to sleep and the clinic organised to have him cremated. Probably a month later, a picture of Bubbles turned up with a thank-you note, a bottle of wine and a box of chocolates. Gifts are an interesting thing in vet science. You can do the most whizz-bang work to save an animal's life and you barely get a thank-you. When the animal dies, however, more often than not you get wine or chocolates or both. I guess people appreciate the compassion that vets show in that time of need, but it remains a mystery to me.

I really treasured Carol's gesture and I hung the picture of Bubbles on the waiting room wall.

A couple of months later, Carol got a new dog, a black cocker spaniel called Snoopy. I thought it was a great idea because it gave her a fresh focus. So I turned up at Carol's house on my next Tuesday run, really happy that we'd be able to continue our personal and professional relationship. I'd missed our weekly chats. Carol opened the door with a big smile, but Snoopy took one look at me, marched to the far side of the room and started making a strange 'huk, huk' noise at me.

'Come in, love. Don't worry about him. He doesn't know you yet. Cup of tea? Biscuit?'

Snoopy was an ex-breeding dog who hadn't received any socialisation or normality in his life. He had been kept solely in a cage for breeding. And he had been 'debarked', which is an illegal procedure whereby the vocal cords are damaged so dogs are less noisy. Instead of a bark, they honk like a seal. The noise is far more annoying than an actual bark and Snoopy seemed to be able to keep it up without respite.

We chatted away and Snoopy didn't stop hukking and honking the whole time. Next visit, same thing. He wouldn't come near me and became pseudo-aggressive if I tried to get anywhere near him. Carol and I couldn't chat with all the noise, so Snoopy got banished to another room which defeated the main purpose of the vet visit. It was awkward. The situation continued for twelve months but my visits became less regular and less enjoyable. One day I was in the clinic flicking through some papers and I noticed that there was a vaccination reminder for Carol. It said Snoopy was two months overdue. This was highly unusual. Carol was normally right on top of all her paperwork.

Something must have happened to her. Worried, I grabbed the phone and rang straight away. She picked up after a couple of rings.

'Oh, Anthony. I feel like such a heel,' she said.

'Why? It doesn't matter if the dog's just a little overdue for its vaccination. We'll fix it up.'

'No, I'm sorry. I've been going to see the new vet that started up out here. He's nearby but I feel so sorry and I'm so sad.'

A rival veterinary practice had opened at the Heads and she said that since we were only there on Tuesdays, it made more sense to go to him.

I felt hurt. The excuse didn't hold water to me because she knew that we'd always go out whenever we were needed. I was certain that the real reason was because Snoopy didn't like me. Behaviourists be damned.

'I'll see you later, then,' I said and hung up, stunned. It was fairly early in my career and I thought that Carol and I had transcended the client–vet relationship. We were friends, weren't we? I had gone many, many times over and above my professional duties and now she'd turned around and gone to see another vet.

The statistics don't lie: the number-one reason that people visit their local vet is because they are the closest vet to their home, quickly followed by the availability of parking. Car trips in a WRX and afternoon teas don't seem to rate a mention.

I continued to drive past her house every Tuesday on the Heads run and I'd wonder whatever became of her, but I've never seen her again nor heard any reports. The picture of Bubbles remained on the wall too, delivering a painful little stab every time I noticed it, but when we renovated a year or two later, it got packed away somewhere and never went back up.

AND JILL CAME TUMBLING AFTER

James

It was the end of summer when John asked me to go out and castrate a colt for an elderly couple. 'I did one there many years ago,' he said. 'It's difficult because it's very hilly and it's hard to find a good spot to do it. You'll be all right, though. You've done loads of these before.'

I arrived at the property to find a lovely old couple who didn't have a clue about horses. The colt was a black Welsh mountain pony that belonged to their son, who'd moved away. All they knew was that they had a horse that needed castrating. When I asked if they could put a halter on him and bring him out of his stable, they looked at me like I was asking them to ride him in the lord of the manor's hunt.

As John had warned me, their house was perched on top of a hill, but it was worse than that. The hill was steeper than I'd imagined and at the bottom of it, 20 metres below, was the motorway, with a barbed-wire fence and a stream in between. There was a lot of potential for things to go wrong.

Where am I going to anaesthetise this horse?

At the house there was a small flat area that dropped away sharply. It was the only spot I could see where we had any hope of doing this. It wasn't so much the operation that was the problem, it was what would happen afterwards. I explained to the couple, 'When you recover a horse, it's very groggy. It attempts to stand and it can stumble a little. That slope you've got there is a big risk. Perhaps we should consider some other options.' They looked at me blankly so I continued. 'Can we go to a neighbour's place, maybe?' I asked.

'No, no. They've been done here before and everything was fine.'

'All right then.' I just had to repeat John's words like a mantra. *You'll be all right. You've done loads of these before.*

Gelding a horse is a difficult procedure. You need to put the colt to sleep with a general anaesthetic. In a dog or cat you do that in a surgical environment where there are other people around to help. But with horses it's done in the field. I coaxed the horse out. His name was Rhys. The old man explained that there had been a Welsh king in the thirteenth century called Rhys the Hoarse, so their son had named this fellow Rhys the Horse.

I drew up the needle of xylazine to sedate Rhys. No problems. I positioned him how I wanted him, then injected the anaesthetic and took control of Rhys's lead rope. A minute or so later, Rhys eased himself to the ground and continued the jerky journey towards a deep, peaceful sleep.

That was the first challenge. The next one was to restrain his leg so that if he started to wake during the surgery he didn't boot me into the middle of next week. With that done, it was time for the procedure. Unlike all the other operations we do where we tie off any veins or arteries that are bleeding, when you castrate a horse you crush the blood vessels with a wonderfully named tool called an emasculator. We can't leave stitches in there because the wound needs to drain and stitches give infections an added place to hide. So the emasculator clamps down on the veins and the spermatic cord. You hold it in place for a minute or two and it seals off the vessels, before the testicles are thrown away.

So I got all my ducks lined up and followed the procedure in the old couple's little flat yard. I gave Rhys the Horse the post-operative injections: tetanus, penicillin and an anti-inflammatory. It all went smoothly. About five minutes after I finished, the horse started to wake. He sat up, looking a bit groggy, but calm. Good. It was exactly what I wanted. He made snorty little noises, gathered himself and looked around to take in his surroundings. He recognised the old couple. Also good. Rhys got up gradually, stumbling slightly. I was holding a lead attached to his halter and was guiding him with the rope when something startled him. I've no idea what it was, but he stumbled to the ground on the edge of the hill. It was that precarious position, 20 metres above the roadway.

Shit, don't move.

Calmly, I talked to him, trying to keep him exactly where he was, but Rhys the Horse had other ideas. He wanted to get up again so I tried to coax him back towards the flat, but he was too big, and I watched, helpless, as he rolled himself off the flat. He only needed one roll to go over, before he started sliding down the hill. He was still quite sedated and groggy from the anaesthetic as he glided downwards. A few metres down, he tried to right himself, stopping momentarily before rolling, sliding, stopping, then taking fright and starting the whole process again. It was a disaster unfolding in slow motion. I scurried behind him but was powerless against his weight until, inevitably, Rhys the Horse reached the barbed-wire fence, coming to rest with his legs underneath the bottom strand of wire just a couple of metres from the stream and a few more from the motorway.

As all horse people know, horses and barbed-wire do not go together, and horses that are panicked, groggy and lying underneath a barbed-wire fence are an especially undesirable combination.

Rhys, however, lay still long enough for me to get to him and put my knees onto his neck to hold him down. 'Can you come quickly and lean on him?' I called urgently to the old chap.

'What can I do?' the wife asked.

'Can you get some wire cutters so we can get him out from under here?'

I'd left a needle and sedatives in my pocket for such an emergency, so while holding him down I drew up a large dose and got it into him. Rhys the Horse calmed down instantly, drifting into a light plane of anaesthesia. By this stage, I was able to lift my gaze sufficiently to realise that cars were going past us at eye level, watching our capers. Fantastic.

Snip. Snip. Snip. Snip. Fortunately the wire cutters were sharp and did the job easily. I don't think I could have handled another disaster.

Now we had the problem of recovering the horse again. I didn't want him to stand up on the hill so we pulled him through the now-cut fence to the narrow strip between the creek and the road. I kept my knees on his neck until he was ready to get up, fearful that any repeat of the episode would result in us entering the nearby stream, or even worse, the horse bolting onto the motorway. Rhys recovered just fine the second time around, and we walked him up the hill and back to his barn. I searched hard for any sign of injury but, much to our amazement, he was completely unharmed. The fence, however, would require some mending.

I got back to the clinic and told John the story. He found it very amusing, especially since it had a happy ending. 'I thought that hill might be a problem,' he said.

Caroline was mortified on my behalf. She only worked with small animals. I think these types of stories reassured her that she had chosen the correct branch of vet science.

I didn't feel too bad about it. Even though it was a bad day, I had foreseen a problem and tried to warn the owners that we should go elsewhere. I was so glad I had. It made me look prophetic. If you tell clients everything is going to be fine and it's not, they can get agitated. But when the outcome is good in the face of adversity, everyone's happy.

At the pub that night, sitting at the bar enjoying the lovely community, someone tapped me on the shoulder. 'Have a good day today?'

'Yes. Yes. Good day.'

'Hmmmm. Had some horse work, did you?'

'Yeeeees.'

'On a hill by any chance?'

My heart was sinking. Word was out. These people knew nothing of the way I'd predicted the disaster, the way I'd overcome it, my neat surgical techniques, nor the happy gelding now enjoying a good night in the stables. Rhys wasn't the only one who'd have to suffer barbs that day.

Another voice came across the bar: 'Hey James, I hear you've taken up steeplechasing over barbed-wire fences …'

And another: 'Oi, James, you leave our Welsh ponies alone …'

'I heard you went for a roll in the hay with a filly.'

'It was a stallion,' I said. 'At least it *was* a stallion before I got a hold of it.'

FAT BOY SLIM

Anthony

Doris Irvine was one of my favourite characters. She was one of those people who might get referred to as 'old Berry'. Wiry, wrinkled and hard of hearing, once she mounted a horse she lost about forty years. Her osteoporotic back and arthritic fingers seemed to straighten in the saddle as she trotted around the yard moving in sync with her old gelding, Slim. You'd never know she was well into her eighties and Slim was well into his twenties.

She rang one day to say that a former show pony she'd bought for her granddaughter to ride was sore. 'Yeah, I think it might be founder,' she said.

Doris knew her horses so I expected she'd be right with her diagnosis. Founder is a disease that horses get if they eat too many readily digestible sugars. It's an inflammatory reaction that occurs everywhere in the body but is most noticeable in the feet. It's very common in ponies because they have adapted to live in poor country where there is little food. Then they come to lush areas like the coast of Australia, get terrifically fat and suffer very badly from founder.

I walked in and the white pony was standing stock-still in what we call the 'sawhorse position' – with her feet extending further out to the front and back than normal, like she was stretching. She was trying to distribute the weight evenly across all four feet because they were equally painful.

The pony's name was Beauty and she looked at me like, 'Cripes, here comes the guy in the green overalls.' She wanted to run, but moving hurt so much she had to stand there. The best she could do was lean away as I approached, her feet anchored in the same spots. At least she was standing. When horses lie down, they are waiting to die.

The horse's hoof is essentially a finger nail. With founder, the membrane between the nail and the foot bone gets excruciatingly inflamed and sore. To get an idea of what Beauty was going through, imagine someone jamming a piece of bamboo underneath your toenail and then asking you to bear all your weight on that nail and walk around. You certainly wouldn't be lining up to go for a run around the paddock.

Beauty was so sore I could not pick up any of her feet. Lifting one off the ground would put more weight on the other three. So no way would she let me budge one. I felt her front left foot on the ground and it was hot with inflammation. I felt the blood vessel running down the side of the leg and it was pounding with all the extra blood flow to the foot. Her pulse was seventy-five beats a minute, which is catastrophically high for a horse.

Beauty was about thirteen years old, and like all show ponies grossly overweight. For whatever reason, the breeders and judges of ponies have determined that their ideal stature is rotund. It's a purely human construct. It's the same for Labradors. People see a Labrador in good shape and they think it's too skinny, but that's just because they are used to seeing obese dogs.

Beauty had a big fat belly and was almost flat across the back with a 'cresting neck', where she had deposited a huge amount of fat in a curve along the top of her neck. I grabbed the area below her mane and it was like a big roll of jelly.

'She's been on too much good feed,' I said across her back.

'What's that, love?' Doris was very hard of hearing.

'She's been eating too much,' I yelled.

'I know she's a bit overweight,' Doris said, 'but I bought her in show condition and now we've had a bit of rain the grass has been jumping up.'

'Doris, this is very bad. It's a really severe case. It must have been going for some time.'

'Gee, I don't know. I only noticed it today.'

I treated Beauty with painkillers and some sedatives to try to control her pain and reduce the inflammation. I wanted to get her into a stable with sand on the floor because that distributes more weight onto the sole of the foot and would ease the burden a little. So I left Doris with instructions to severely restrict Beauty's diet and that when the painkillers kicked in, to try to get her to the sandy stable.

I called at the end of the day and Doris said they'd got the horse halfway across the yard, but then couldn't get her any further.

Next morning, I went back and Beauty was still there, halfway to the sandy stable. She had all the same symptoms but she was sitting now. She couldn't cop it any longer and we couldn't get her to stand. This was probably the best thing to relieve her distress but it made the prognosis poor. I got down on my knees and gave her more intravenous painkillers and sedatives and left more painkillers for Doris to administer. I had a bad feeling that this wasn't going to end well. Severe inflammation like this can cause the tendon up the back of the leg – the equivalent of our Achilles tendon – to pull the pedal bone so hard that it rotates through the sole of the hoof. And that's the end of the horse.

I called Doris the next morning, the third day I'd been on the case, because I wasn't confident she was treating it as seriously as I thought it

needed. I suspected she thought it was just an ordinary case of founder –
'We'll give the horse some painkillers and she'll be right.'

'How's Beauty going?' I asked. 'Has she got any better?' I was
expecting Doris to say she was terrible and why wasn't there something
more I could do. But no.

'Yes, yes, Anthony,' she said. 'She's much better now. She's almost
back to normal.'

'Oh … great. That's amazing.' I didn't quite believe it. I couldn't
see how it could have got better overnight.

'Thank you for everything you've done. We're really happy and the
horse looks like it's on the mend.'

'That's great.'

'Ever since her front foot fell off yesterday afternoon, she's just been
so much better.'

'What do you mean her foot fell off? A bit of its nail?'

'No, no, her hoof fell off. And now she seems quite relieved. It's
going to get better.'

I'd never heard of such a thing. 'Okay, Doris, I'm coming straight
out. Don't go anywhere.' I jumped in the car and sped over. When I
arrived, I didn't bother pulling on my overalls like I normally would.
'Where's Beauty?' I asked Doris, my anxiety clearly showing.

'What's wrong? She's fine. She's over there. What do you need to
do for her?'

'I think we might need to put her down.'

'Huh? Why?'

'Well, from what you described, I think she's walking around on
raw bone. She must be in excruciating pain.'

As we headed towards the shed, Doris touched my shoulder and
pointed to a post. 'There's her foot.' On the top of the post was the
whole hoof, empty like a cup.

Extraordinary. I couldn't believe it. Beauty had made it to the sandy stable now. When we reached her she was standing, so Doris might have been right when she said she was in less pain than the day before, but the rest of her didn't appear any better. It looked to me that she was in just as much pain walking around on raw bone as she had been on her inflamed hooves. Her heart rate was up around ninety. She was sweating and really uncomfortable. Her eyes, bulging and white, were wild.

And there was no way she was going to move any further.

'Can't you see how much pain this horse is in?'

'Oh yeah, but I think she's on the improve.'

I gathered that the inflammation of the membrane that held the hoof to the bone had caused it to give way, allowing the hoof to just fall off. You could never nurse that animal back to health. You'd have to suspend it off the ground for six months of non-weight-bearing while the nail grew back, if it ever did. If it happened in a human you could manage it without a problem, but this was 450 kilograms that wouldn't lie down in a bed. It just wasn't feasible, even for the most valuable horse.

There was a famous case in the states where they kept a multi-million dollar trotter in a float tank while its leg repaired. After a long rehab, they led it out of the tank and as its full weight came back on its limbs it promptly broke its leg. The bones had gone soft after so long without bearing any load.

I put Beauty down immediately. I didn't need a lot of help. She didn't move. Even if she wanted to she wouldn't have been able to lift a leg to kick me. I just needed to find the jugular. We don't like the owners holding the horse during euthanasia because it's always a bit unpredictable as to where and how the horse will fall. Beauty just crumpled at the knees and fell to her side.

Doris was okay with it. She'd seen a lot of horses come and go in her more than eighty years, but she was a little upset with me for letting her know I thought she'd let this one go too far without calling me.

'If anything like that happens again, you've got to call me immediately,' I said.

'Well, if any of the others' feet fall off, I'll be sure to give you a whistle.'

CHAVS AND CHAV-NOTS

James

I loved Wales and would have stayed longer if the opportunity was there, but John and Caroline had a permanent replacement coming in. The farewell party started at the pub. They all dressed in what they thought was Australian national costume – there were lots of shorts and thongs, though the Welsh called them flip-flops. I was forced to wear a bizarre form of Welsh national dress – a barbecue apron and an inflatable sheep. The party headed back to my place and kicked on. It spewed out into the communal vet areas and red wine found its way onto the carpet, a gate found its way off its hinges, and a coffee table found its way back into its original flat-pack state. I didn't find my way into bed till 7 a.m., and didn't find my way out of it till 3 p.m.

The problem was that I was due in London the following morning for a flight to Spain and a holiday with some vet friends. Before I could even think about packing, I had to fix the gate, rebuild the coffee table and scrub the carpet till my arms could scrub no more, sweat dripping from my nose into the suds. It was horrendous to do all this while suffering a severe hangover. But there was no choice. I couldn't leave John and Caroline's place a mess and I had to catch that flight. So I cleaned and packed till 4 a.m., had an hour's sleep, made a stiff coffee, then drove the Ford Fiesta I had bought from Caroline's mother hard down the grey motorways to London airport.

There were twelve Sydney Uni vets working in the UK and someone had organised for us to meet up and go to San Sebastian. What a great choice. It's an impossibly beautiful town that looks a bit like Rio de Janeiro; surrounded by imposing mountains with high rises on the beach but cobblestoned back alleys further inland, where behind every door hides a tiny bar. We moved from bar to bar where they line up the pintxo (the Basque equivalent of tapas), on the counter and you eat and drink to your heart's content. No money changes hands till you tell them what you've consumed as you're leaving. There's no question of telling fibs. All the barkeepers are dark and mysterious types who look like Basque separatist hard-men.

We danced and shouted and had a wonderful time and all the while I was aware of this tall and beautiful presence. Her name was Ronnie and she was travelling with a school friend who was one of the vets from the year below us. We moved to a little bar with nets and jugs hanging from the ancient rafters and at last I got a chance to sit next to this girl.

Someone had ordered white wine and Ronnie had a glass that I noticed she'd hardly touched. 'Not much of a drinker?' I said, seizing my opportunity to make small talk.

'No, I love a drink,' she said. 'It's just terrible white wine.' I ridiculed her for such snobbery. I'd never met a wine that couldn't be put away. 'Do you want me to finish it for you?'

She said okay, with a doubtful look on her face.

Before it had even passed my tongue it was just about coming back through my nostrils. It was, indeed, clearly the worst wine ever manufactured outside a vinegar factory. She found it hilarious and we spent the rest of the night and early morning drinking and dancing and going from pintxo bar to pintxo bar. She must have seen something beneath my dusty exterior because we made tentative arrangements to catch up back in the UK when she got back from doing a lap around Europe.

After Spain, I returned to the UK and a new job in a place called Wisbech (pronounced Wizz Beach). Going through the locum agency's job list, I'd seen this vacancy in Cambridgeshire and had visions of universities and punting on the river in flannels. I arrived on the train and my new boss, Mr Paton, picked me up and took me for a quick look around the old Georgian heart of the town. It lay on the River Nene and was quite striking.

'I'll take you to the flat we've rented for you,' Mr Paton said. We proceeded to drive through drab streets of council flats and teens pushing prams. 'It's probably best you don't go out after 7 p.m.,' he said.

'Oh yeah?'

'Things can get a little dangerous. The rougher elements of town tend to emerge from under their rocks.'

My flat was in a small gated community, beside a church and above a Subway. The smell of baking bread permeated the unit. When I turned on the television news that first night, late in the bulletin there was a story about police initiatives to curb crime in Wisbech because it had the third highest crime rate of any postcode in the UK. That was troubling. Later that night I heard a fight outside my window in the alley between my building and the church. I was to learn that the alleyway was a favoured venue not only for pugilism but also for romance and commerce, i.e. sex and drug deals.

And just to set the scene a little further, a doctor later told me that 22 per cent of the population had chlamydia and there was also a very high AIDS rate.

For all that, Mr Paton ran a really good practice. It was a tight ship, with a good variety of work. Even though there were elements of urban slum, it didn't take long to drive out onto the Fens and into some of the best agricultural land in Britain.

The urban clientele was – how should I say? – 'different'. In Australia some might call them bogans. In the UK they were called chavs. I couldn't find an entry for chavs in my *Manual of Exotic Pets*, but the Oxford English Dictionary defines 'chav' as an informal pejorative used to refer to a type of anti-social, uncultured youth, who wears a lot of flashy jewellery, white trainers, a baseball cap and fake designer clothes. Chavettes, the female of the species, expose a lot of midriff.

Chav dogs were almost exclusively Staffordshire bull terriers. Chavs love Staffies. They're pretty much their emblem. And all these dogs had horrendous problems, which the chavs had no money to fix. That's one enduring memory. The other is that whenever the temperature went above 20 degrees, it was seen as an invitation to take your shirt off in order to display your fat, white belly covered in tattoos. I dreaded the heat, and found myself pining for the cold of Wales. And not because I had no tattoos on my belly.

I'd walk into the waiting room and there would be three big guys; covered in ink, no shirts, all with Staffies at heel. It was like there'd been a council order. A lot of the dogs had skin problems from fleas that hadn't been treated properly. I'd say, 'Tyson here has fleas, that's why he's scratching so much.' And they'd say, 'Oh, is m'dog scratching?'

It was a challenge.

The other thing that will stay with me was the landscape. The Fens were eerily flat. If it wasn't for the odd tree, you'd swear you could see forever. It's all reclaimed sea floor so, like the Netherlands, is criss-crossed by canals and dotted with windmills. And, like the Netherlands, it is flat, flat, flat.

There was no risk of your horse rolling down the hill after castration here. Mr Paton told me that there were people who couldn't cope with the flatness. It would freak them out and they'd head for the hills. 'But it also messes with the animals,' he said. 'I did a pre-purchase examination on a horse a few years back. This was a ten-year-old horse that I knew well. It was quiet and in sound condition. I signed off all the paperwork and the horse was bought by someone who took it away to another district up north. A few weeks later, the people who bought it rang me and said, "We're not very happy. You did the pre-purchase examination and you stated that it is a quiet horse with an even temperament. We cannot get this horse to leave the yard. It bucks and kicks. It's fine in the dressage arena but if we take it out it goes crazy."

'I had a pal up there who I asked to go and look at it for me and he confirmed what they said. This was very strange because I knew it was a good horse. They ended up taking the horse down the hill to another place and it was fine. This horse had lived all its life on the Fens. It had never seen a hill, and certainly wasn't about to start walking on one. They had to re-educate the horse that hills weren't going to kill it. I was very relieved that I wasn't going to get sued for a negligent pre-purchase agreement.'

A month or so after I got to Wisbech, Ronnie returned from Europe and came up to visit me. It was a fairly brave step for her, but she ended up staying about a week. We laughed a lot about the funny little place we'd found ourselves in. That's the beauty of working your way around the country. This was a view of the UK the ordinary tourist didn't get to see – the have-nots.

I remember one night we did a mercy dash to Tesco after midnight for some supplies. We were amazed at the number of people who were there filling baskets with Coke and chips. Ronnie summed it up best: 'If you ever want to feel good about your weight, just go to Wisbech Tesco at 1 a.m.'

CUSHION'S DISEASE

Anthony

'There's something drastically wrong with Dolly,' Kathy Sabel said, following me through the unusually crowded reception area with her fluffy white dog cradled in her arms.

'What's wrong?' I asked, dodging a little yellow puddle at the feet of a panting bull terrier.

'She's got a *huge* appetite,' Kathy said, doing her best to emphasise the vastness of it. 'Yet she still seems to be losing weight.'

'Okay, what are you feeding her?' I asked, thinking that the main reason dogs have big appetites is they don't get fed enough.

'A cup of dried food in the morning and a cup in the afternoon, plus some tuna and bits and pieces. That's what she's eaten all her life and now she's got this huge appetite and I weighed her today and she's a kilo lighter than she was last time. She was eight and a half, and now she's only seven and a half.'

'Well, dogs are gluttons,' I said. 'They don't have an off button with their appetite.'

'But I got home from work yesterday and Dolly had broken into the pantry and she'd eaten two full boxes of Tiny Teddy biscuits and she was so bloated she couldn't move. Her belly was sticking out like a balloon.'

'Did you do that Dolly Sabel?' I said, addressing the fluffy white shih tzu-Maltese cross now sitting on the table in the consult room.

'So I was pretty horrified about that,' Kathy continued, 'but then Lachlan got home from work and he always feeds her as soon as he comes in. Before I realised he'd done it, he'd scooped out her usual cup of dog food. Dolly took one look at it, peeled herself off the ground and waddled over like a great fat slug and demolished the lot.'

Lachlan and Kathy were a lovely couple who owned the antique shop in town. They really loved this dog and I knew they were pretty sensible about its care.

'Was this a one-off?'

'No, she broke into Lachlan's mum's room when she was down for Christmas. Dolly ate all the soap in her toiletry bag and then she ate all the buttons off a dress his mum had laid out to wear that night.'

Kathy was on a roll now. 'Then we took her down to the beach the other day and she started eating bluebottles. They were stinging her. You could see it was uncomfortable by the way she was shaking her head and pawing at her mouth, but she kept going. She'd run a bit further and find another and eat it.'

The fact Dolly was losing weight despite all this food intake indicated there was something wrong. I had my suspicions as to what it was, but didn't want to say too much till I could be sure. 'We'll take some blood tests and have a look at her.'

We did the tests and they came back showing Dolly had some very elevated liver enzymes, which gave me a further clue. It didn't appear to be an actual liver disease because her symptoms didn't match that, so I suspected a separate problem that was affecting the liver as a secondary issue. There's a disease called Cushing's disease – where a tumour on the adrenal gland or the pituitary gland causes the adrenal gland to secrete too much cortisol. This in turn leads to, among other things, a huge appetite, a huge thirst and a lot of urine production.

I asked the Geoffs about it and they said they'd never seen a case of it in Berry before. I ordered in the hormone that is used to diagnose Cushing's, did the test and the readings came back ballistically high, confirming my suspicion.

Kathy and Lachlan both came in to talk about it. They were very concerned. Their children had grown up and moved out, so Dolly was the centre of their lives.

Lachlan, tall with a thick moustache, didn't speak a lot but his words were considered. Kathy, striking to look at with her pale complexion under an always-made-up face, was more inclined to speak quickly. You knew what she was thinking immediately she thought it.

I explained the prognosis to them as best I could but it was difficult to get across what lay ahead. They kept calling it Cushion's disease. The treatment back then was particularly dangerous. The only drug we had was mitotane and it was more like chemotherapy than normal medicine. If you overdose a dog it can die from a lack of cortisone (Addison's disease).

'You have to give her just enough over three to seven days to partially kill the adrenal gland to the point where things are brought back into balance,' I said. 'If I prescribe her too much she will die. If I get it right, she will be back to normal and then we just have to give her a dose every week or two to keep her in balance.'

'So you just need to give the right amount of *poison*?' Kathy asked.

'How do you know what the right amount is?' Lachlan said.

'Yes, it is poison and, well, I don't know what the right amount is. That's the difficulty. You'll have to give it to her for a few days at home then test her again.'

'And what is the alternative if we do nothing?'

'If you don't treat her, she'll lose the ability to maintain muscle. So she may have heart problems. She'll become pot-bellied, lose a lot of hair, and waste away despite a voracious appetite. She might become aggressive and start stealing food off tables, off people, off children. But eventually she'll fade away and die.'

How do you convince someone to give their dog poison for an uncertain outcome at considerable cost?

But Lachlan and Kathy were great. They wanted to pursue this to the end. We treated Dolly with the mitotane for three days then got her back in for another test. The results came back the next day showing we hadn't treated her for quite long enough so we dosed her for one more day before we pulled back. We got Dolly's 'Cushion's' disease well under control and she returned to a happy life. A few years later, a safer drug came around, but things were so well controlled by the mitotane that we decided not to risk a change.

It would have been three years later, when Dolly was about twelve years old, that she was brought back in, really sick and bedraggled. She'd lost a lot of teeth, she was smelly, her ears were bad, and her eyesight was failing. It didn't take more than a cursory look for me to determine that this was the end of the line for Dolly Sabel.

Cushing's is, ultimately, a cancer. Most dogs with Cushing's don't live long enough for the cancer to start causing other problems. Dolly was a tough dog but now it appeared her condition had caught up with her. When I tried to stand her up on the examination table, she collapsed, making a groaning noise.

So we had the big talk. Everyone was upset. I said that Dolly had had a great run, living with Cushing's so long, but that it always got them in the end. It was time to think about Dolly's best interests. Kathy was very distressed but, like a lot of women in that position, remained rational at the same time. She asked a few questions through the tears. Lachlan looked at me as if to say, I'm only holding it together because I don't think there is room for the two of us to lose it.

Lachlan was getting quieter the longer we talked. I've noticed with a lot of men that they'll come in with no emotion – 'Everything's under control here. Ignore my wife. She's very attached to Fluffy. We'll handle this man-to-man. We'll go out the back, shoot it then go have a beer.' They don't actually say that, of course, but you get the drift. But when the blokes crack, they really go to pieces. And here's the thing: they always crack.

Lachlan was saying nothing now, striving to maintain the strong outward persona, but his upper lip was quivering. Kathy was crying, but talking. She was the one who took charge. 'Look, we know we're going to have to put Dolly to sleep; we just want one more night with her. We know she's in distress and discomfort but we need one more night to deal with this.'

So we put Dolly on a drip and sent her home with painkillers. Lachlan and Kathy hoped that Dolly would pass away quietly in her sleep but I knew that dogs don't go quietly. I was fully expecting a call in the middle of the night.

Despite my reservations about letting Dolly go home, the Geoffs had drilled into me that there was no right or wrong way. If a client had very strong feelings in one direction, and there were no obvious welfare issues, it was best to go along with them. The Geoffs had over sixty years of veterinary experience between them and, despite my misgivings, they were my mentors and I accepted their views.

Still, I didn't think that Dolly would see out the night, or that Kathy and Lachlan were well equipped to see her die at home.

First thing the next morning I called their home expecting to hear that Dolly was dead or that they wanted me to come straight out to put her down.

Kathy, however, was peculiarly bright and effusive. 'I'm going to bring her in straight away,' she said.

'Okay, we're free now.'

I went and got the Lethabarb, gathering my gear for the sad job at hand then, minutes later, Dolly trotted through the door, looked at me, barked, ate something, drank from a bowl and proceeded to sniff around the waiting-room chairs.

'We sat up with her for most of the night,' Kathy explained. 'She was very quiet all night, we thought we'd lost her numerous times; however, she kept breathing and would open an eyelid when we called her name. We both fell asleep sometime around 4 a.m. and when we woke up we couldn't believe our eyes. Dolly was trotting around the house like nothing was wrong. She had even chewed her drip line out as if to say, "I don't need that any more."'

I have no idea what caused her illness and no idea how she got better. But she did. It was a resurrection. Dolly Sabel lived for another two full years. Just fine.

I learnt an important lesson that day. If I had based my decision purely on my medical training, Dolly would have been euthanased. But because I listened to the client, nature took its course and surprised me. You don't learn everything at university. Sometimes you have to listen to the people around you.

A POSH PADDLEPOP

James

The Wisbech clinic had a loyal employee, Ricky Watling, who'd been there for twenty years. Now, while Ricky had a mild intellectual disability, he worked diligently at cleaning the cages, helping to hold animals and doing all the little jobs that needed doing around the place. He must have been in his late thirties and he'd spent all those years accumulating an encyclopaedic knowledge of the Liverpool Football Club. Because I was male, he pretty much assumed that I'd be equally fascinated by Liverpool FC and all things related to English soccer. He'd talk about it all day every day, which was fine by me, but everyone else was like, 'Please, Ricky, shut up.'

Ricky was also a keen observer of patterns. He knew, for instance, that if Ronnie was in town, we'd go to the pub for lunch, and he also knew our favourite places for dinner. Lo and behold, he would always turn up. As we tucked into our meals, we'd see his dumpy frame heading towards us with his very short dark hair and see-through pale skin. We'd have to laugh. It was all part of the fun. He was a real character.

But Ricky had a bit of a target on his back. He had the ability to sometimes upset people by being not as socially aware as others. One night we were at the pub and he must have said something because one of the chavs wanted to fight him.

We drank up and grabbed our jackets: 'Come on, Ricky. We'll walk you home.'

As we strolled back to his place we chatted about his life. 'You live with your parents?'

'Yeah, yeah. My grandparents, my parents, my brother and my sister. We all live in the house together.'

'What do your grandparents do?'

'Nothing, they've never had a job.'

'And your parents?'

'No, never had a job neither.'

'And your brother?'

'No, he don't work. Who'd give him a job?'

So Ricky, with his intellectual disability, was the only one in three generations who'd had a job. It didn't seem to me that Ricky thought of his employed state as being anything out of the ordinary. He wanted to turn up each day in order to help animals and to talk about Liverpool FC. The fact no one else in his family worked was totally normal; he'd just decided to go a different way.

Wisbech certainly was different. No more so than the day Mary Goodacre burst into the clinic with a border collie cross in her arms. I'd seen a bit of her and the dog, Posh, in recent weeks, and my predecessors had looked after her before that. Mary, a slightly stumpy woman, came through the door like her greasy black hair was on fire. 'Quick, quick. You've got to see Posh. Where's the vet? She's dying.'

For Mary, everything was an emergency. So we weren't as hurried as we otherwise might have been.

Posh had horrendous diabetes, which Mary had been unable to treat. I gathered that Mary suffered a mild intellectual disability and, no matter how much she loved Posh, she just hadn't been able to keep up with the rigorous treatment. She hadn't fed the dog regularly enough, nor had she kept to the tight schedule of insulin injections. Treating diabetes sporadically is dangerous.

Posh couldn't walk now. She looked up to me from Mary's arms with sad, slow eyes sunken in their sockets. She was impossibly skinny. I examined her and it appeared that Mary was right. I diagnosed diabetic ketoacidosis, which I explained to Mary was the end stage of diabetes when the animal is crashing and basically attempting to die. Because Posh couldn't metabolise glucose, her body had started to feed off the protein in her muscles, which left them wasted and thin. Typically, dogs can survive like this for a while, but eventually an infection comes along and everything falls to pieces. That's where Posh was at now: dehydrated, weak, very skinny and moribund.

As gently as possible, I said, 'Posh has reached this point despite your very best efforts and so I think it might be time to put her to sleep.'

Much discussion ensued with Mary speaking in her short, urgent sentences, and me doing my best not to sound like I was blaming her.

Posh was getting on too. I presumed she had been a pup when the Spice Girls had had their first hits, so she was probably about eleven or twelve. Even if Mary could have given her the best care, Posh wasn't going to live much longer. It took a long time to explain this to Mary and to have her understand what we needed to do.

'Yes. We must help Posh,' she said, eventually. 'You've got to stop her pain.' And so it was with much sadness all round that we put Posh to sleep for the very last time and Mary waddled out with tears in her eyes.

Two days later, however, I heard a commotion out in the waiting room and heard Mary asking for me. I came out into the reception area with some trepidation as she rushed over to see me, not quite leaving me the usual buffer zone of personal space.

'I really want to see Posh,' she said. 'I really need to see her.'

'Okay. Why do you want to see Posh?'

'I need to know that she's really dead.'

'Okay. I can get Posh out for you. But you realise that she's been in cold storage for several days? She might not be looking that nice.'

'Yes, yes. I just need to see her. It's for me own mental well-being.'

'Okay, I'll go and arrange that. You just wait here.' So I went to the freezer out the back. Unfortunately, after Posh died she had urinated profusely post-mortem within the bag in which she was stored. The bag was put into the freezer on a slight angle and all the urine had run to the end where her head was, before it froze. So Posh's head was now encased in an enormous golden iceblock in an awful contorted position. *What do I do now?*

There was nothing for it but to grab some surgical instruments and start chipping away in much the same way one might use a hammer and chisel. Immediately the edges started to thaw, the awful smell of deep-yellow urine from dehydrated dog filled my nostrils. I was screwing up my nose while banging at the weird icy dog-pop. My colleagues looked at me like I was demented.

'You don't want to know,' was the best I could offer them.

'Nah, what are you doing?' Ricky persisted.

I told him. He scratched his chin from a safe distance. 'Nah, I wouldn't do it like that. You need a chisel.'

'Thanks, Ricky. Can you get one and give me a hand?'

'Nah, we ain't got a chisel. But that's what you need. Or a hairdryer. Maybe a heat gun?'

It took about twenty minutes of hard work. I was sweating. But I'd got the ice off and managed to make Posh look a little less horrific, positioning her nicely and wrapping her in fresh towels. Still it wasn't pretty. I figured, however, there was nothing more I could do short of a complete mortician's makeover.

'If you could come this way, Mary,' I said in a gentle voice like I imagine undertakers might use. I led her in, full of apprehension. 'Now, she has been in cold storage and she doesn't look her best,' I said.

Mary looked at the dog for perhaps two seconds. 'Yep, that's definitely Posh. She's definitely dead. Thanks, James.'

She turned around and walked away, nonchalant.

I suppose she needed to lock that one away in her own mind. It wasn't about grieving. I'm sure I could have left Posh's head in the ice and Mary wouldn't have cared. I don't know, maybe she thought we were stealing her dog. One thing I did know was that people deal with death in many different ways. Whenever we put a dog to sleep we explain that we can do it however the owner wants. You can be with the dog. You can leave the dog with us. You can pick it up afterwards to bury yourself. You can have us send it to a pet crematorium. However, we never, ever offer to have their heads encased in a golden iceblock.

MANNING THE FORT

Anthony

There was an interesting dynamic between the two Geoffs. Geoff Scarlett was a really big man. Thick-set and outgoing, he had a big personality and was a social kind of guy. Geoff Manning could also be like that sometimes, but it was underneath a few layers of complexity. He was, essentially, reserved and quiet – characteristics that could be perceived by those who didn't know him as gruffness.

Geoff Scarlett was five or six years Geoff Manning's junior. I always assumed that when Geoff Manning retired I'd buy him out and go into partnership with Geoff Scarlett, which was part of the reason I'd chosen to come to Berry in the first place. But one day I overheard a snippet of conversation between them suggesting that Geoff Scarlett might be leaving. It left me in a bit of a limbo, not knowing what was going on, but eventually Geoff Scarlett came and told me.

'Look, I'm retiring,' he said, explaining that his right wrist was giving him hell and he couldn't continue to work. Among other things, he'd aggravated it lifting cows' tails during the tuberculosis eradication program in the 1980s. They'd had to go around to all the farms and give every single cow a small dose of intradermal tuberculosis in the fold under the tail. Two days later, they'd gone back and lifted each cow's tail to see if a bleb had formed. If it had, the cow had tuberculosis and she'd have to be culled. The incidence of tuberculosis was minimal in this area but it was a national program so no cow could be missed. He tested 30,000 cows. Now he was the final casualty of bovine tuberculosis. 'I'm a cull,' he said. 'You'll have to talk to Geoff about what's happening with the practice.'

After a brief discussion, Geoff Manning explained that he was buying Geoff Scarlett out but that I'd be looked after. A year later, in 2008, Geoff Manning sold me half the practice at a very reasonable price. Geoff and I went on to have a fantastic partnership. He was like a father figure to me. I had a great relationship with his family, who all treated me like I was one of them. I was the same age as Geoff's children too. In fact, his daughter, Georgia, was born the day after me. Geoff was caring and always supportive, and increasingly over the years I got him on side with my ambitions for the practice.

I wanted to open a branch clinic in Kangaroo Valley, but I knew Geoff would be reluctant because he'd had thirty years to do it himself and hadn't. The two Geoffs had once run a branch practice at Shoalhaven Heads out of someone's garage, but once council got wind of it they let it lapse and just reverted to the regular Tuesday run out there. Then that Carol-stealing competitor opened a practice at the Heads, cutting our grass. We considered the Heads to be our turf, just like we considered Kangaroo Valley to be ours.

I thought we couldn't let that happen again. I was determined to open a practice in Kangaroo Valley. It was a prime spot for some young vet to come along and hang his shingle … and that young vet was going to be me.

We had dropped from a three-vet practice to two, but I wasn't keen to put anyone else on for a while. Like anyone who buys a business, I was driven by fear. Geoff and I were working much harder, but turnover and profitability were up. I wanted to keep it going with the Kangaroo

Valley expansion. Eventually I talked him around with the idea that we'd start on a very small, low-cost scale. We opened for business in one of our nurse's garages for just one day a week.

I'd go over there at 7 a.m. and there was so much to do I wouldn't get back to Berry till 3 p.m. or 4 p.m. We realised we were on to a pretty good thing. So we just built it up slowly. I had to prove that each step of the way wasn't a waste of money and that it made business sense. As we went along, Geoff became easier to convince because the ideas were working.

We toiled five days one week and five and a half days the next, and we each did every second night on-call during the week. Whoever had the weekend would do Friday night to Monday night. So when the weekday rotation gave you Tuesday as well, you ended up doing five nights straight on-call. You have to have done on-call work to know what that's like. It's not about being busy, it's the fact you are waiting for the phone to ring; not being able to switch off and go for a run or a surf or even to Kiama because you have to be within a certain distance of the practice. Work dictates your life and is partly why it is difficult to get young vets to the country. Most of the city practices switch their phones to 24-hour emergency centres. You can't do that in a country practice because the distances are often too great.

After a while, I figured that the practice needed a facelift. It was a major undertaking to convince Geoff to spruce up the place, since it was working just fine as it was. I talked him around but didn't tell him something else I had in mind.

One day when Geoff was out I saw all the nurses, Trish, Marie and Rebecca, standing at the front desk. 'What would you think about having a fish tank here?' I asked, gesticulating like a game-show hostess. Their chorus of assent indicated I was on a winner. 'I've always wanted a fish tank in the practice,' I said. 'It's a nice finishing touch, a soothing noise and it's pretty. But Geoff's going to go through the roof. He's going to hate it. So I need you guys to be a part of this. When I put the idea to him, you've got to chip in and say what a fantastic idea it is. Okay?'

'Okay.'

A few days later I judged the mood to be good and I briefed the girls. 'Today's the day I tell him about the fish tank. Are you ready?'

'Yep. We're pumped.'

Geoff appeared from the consult room, all smiles, as he saw his favourite client, Caz Holt, to the front door with her dog. My moment had come. 'Geoff, you know, I think what would really finish this renovation off perfectly would be a nice fish tank here in the waiting room.'

Watching his face, it was like that thing mimes do when they pass their hand downwards over their face and it goes from a smile to a frown.

But Trish, Marie and Rebecca chipped in perfectly before he could get a word in.

'That'd be fantastic.'

'What a ripper idea.'

'Wouldn't it look great over there?'

It was all to no avail. I've never seen someone go so close to exploding. 'No, no ... no, no, no, no ... no, no, no, no, no.' He turned and walked out, still muttering. 'No, no, no, no, no ... no, no, no, no, no.'

Well that was that, I thought. But half an hour later he returned. 'Actually, Anthony, I think it's probably quite a good idea to get that fish tank. I think we should get one.'

As it turned out, James Turk, the mechanic next door, used to own a pet shop. I was chatting to him about it and he said that he'd had a tank in his shop that just seemed to attract people to it. 'I couldn't sell it because it was such a great tank,' James had said. 'I've still got it but I'm not using it. I'll tell you what, I'll give it to you in exchange for a big bag of dog food.'

Geoff, needless to say, was stoked with the deal.

IN A TWIST

James

Ronnie and I were growing increasingly fond of each other, enjoying all the excitement of new romance locked up in our little love fortress in Wisbech. Ronnie, however, worked in human resources in the financial services sector and there weren't many jobs for that sort of thing on the Fens. As winter darkened the countryside and the global financial crisis dimmed employment prospects, she managed to find a job in London. My job was more transportable so I went back to the locum agency and found a spot at a practice in a place called Beckenham, 16 kilometres south of the Tower of London.

It was a practice that largely ran on locums. It was owned by the most eccentric man I've ever met. His name was Clinton 'CJ' Jefferies. He was in his sixties and had run the practice for a long time without doing too much veterinary work. He basically just employed Australian locums and focused his energies on managing us. It's amazing how many vets I meet now who worked for CJ. He did still love to operate and he had some quirky techniques. I remember him showing me how he repaired cruciates, using a slice of skin from the animal in question. CJ said that this was how all cruciates were to be done in the practice. So I said that I'd leave that to him, then. Years later, I was discussing different techniques for cruciate repair with my boss back in Sydney and when I mentioned this method he turned around and said, 'CJ! You must have worked for CJ too!'

CJ looked like a mad professor, bald on top with white hair encircling his bare dome, and a white handlebar moustache drooping down his cheeks. He got around in socks and sandals. You always heard him coming because he had so many keys jangling from his belt in a football-sized cluster.

CJ was also a hoarder. Out the back he had sheds full of stuff. When he finished filling one, he built another. There was a whole office you couldn't get into because of all the paper in there. Only the clinic cats knew the way in and they'd use it as their personal toilet.

He loved printers. One of his principal shed-fillers was printers long since made redundant by the march of technology, mostly in their unopened boxes. He'd get a good deal on them and buy four. He was always going to the hardware store and buying eight of whatever he didn't need.

You couldn't help liking CJ but his practice was as eccentric as he was. We did the on-call work for nineteen other clinics at night. One of us would be on call and you'd do at least four or five jobs per night. It meant that the clinic was overstaffed during the day but very busy at night for whoever was on. Sometimes you'd work right through to dawn and never see your bed.

Ronnie and I moved into a 4-metre by 6-metre flat above the clinic. We decided to renovate it, and when I went looking for tools, I found four 18-volt power drills in their boxes and a couple of electric sanders. I was sorted. CJ was obviously hoarding them for a post-power-tools Armageddon.

We recarpeted the flat and painted it, installing a new kitchen and buying new furniture, all for a grand cost of £1200. One of the features that Ronnie and I didn't like was that the shower cubicle was covered in lino. CJ had a love of lino that bordered on obsession. Everything was lino-ed, including the lowest metre and a half of all the clinic walls. So when the tray at the bottom of the shower was changed years previously and there was a gap between the tray and the tiles, it was no problem for CJ; he simply lino-ed the shower cubicle – no more leaks. I pulled that lino off along with thirty years of muck and vet DNA and re-tiled it at the bottom.

CJ followed a unique business model (not one that has taken off, for some reason), and communication was a common problem exacerbated by the transient workforce. CJ's answer for this was signs. He loved signs and lamination and fonts more than he loved printers. I once did a count of the signs in the darkroom where we developed X-rays. This is a room without any light. You couldn't read anything in there, but there were eleven signs. In the waiting room, where there was plenty of illumination, there were forty-eight. In the operating theatre there was one: 'Do not pull this lever too hard or the window will SHATTER', and 'shatter' was in a font like broken glass.

Every sign was on slightly different coloured paper. He'd put tags on things saying 'Do Not Lose' or 'Do Not Drop' on an expensive phone. He'd put signs on the back of tubes: 'You must label your tubes.' 'You must label your labels.' It was overwhelming. No one read the signs. There were too many. You mightn't see CJ all week, but some problem would bring him back with a new sign. 'Make sure you do NOT leave the CATS here!'

Any problem that arose would be greeted with, 'Well I don't know what more I can do. I've already made a sign about it, but I'll have to make a bigger one.' He would then disappear for three or four hours before emerging with a new sign to get some feedback on the font choice.

There was so much sign saturation that one staff member began removing a sign a day, yet after a month there was no discernible difference.

I worked there for quite some time and ended up taking on some of the day-to-day management of the business for him. It was great experience and I learnt a lot about how to run a practice, as well as how not to. I tried negotiating better deals on how he bought his drugs and how he managed the staff and the pricing structure. I wanted to do it because I liked living there but found myself so frustrated by how it all worked. I thought that if I fixed a few things I might be less frustrated.

Beckenham was like Sydney's Upper North Shore with big houses and leafy gardens. The cricket club where I played and made some lifelong friends was right over the road. But council housing is spread evenly across London so there was quite a melting pot out there too. Next to Beckenham was Catford, one of the rougher bits of London, famous for being a bus depot. We always said that in London you never had to travel too far to get stabbed – or get a good curry.

The leafy suburban side of things was interesting. Cats were much more prevalent in the UK than in Australia. Once again I saw a lot of pocket pets and kept my trusty exotics manual handy. There were still a lot of Staffies, but mixed in with some different breeds: flat-coated retrievers, a British breed of hunting dog; Labrador retrievers; giant Leonbergers; and French bulldogs. But from a veterinary point of view what stood out was the nights. Because we covered for nineteen clinics, we were getting most of the emergency work for South-East London. Dogs hit by cars, busses hit by Rottweilers, blocked cats, poisoned rabbits.

All the clinics had their phones forwarded to us and the nurse downstairs would take the call. She'd phone up to me: 'There's a dog coming in in twenty minutes. It's been hit by a car.'

'Okay, can you get the oxygen ready? Get the X-ray ready and a drip set up.'

I'd get out of bed and dress myself then lie down on the bed and go back to sleep because often people wouldn't turn up. Maybe the dog died already or they just decided the dog didn't need treatment any more. So I'd close my eyes until the nurse rang again to say they'd arrived. It was only a ten-second run down the stairs to the clinic.

You could almost set your watch to the arrival of dogs with twisted stomachs. It usually happened a bit after 10 p.m. The dog had been fed its dinner, maybe it had eaten too much or drunk too much on top of dried food. Then it had a romp before bed while its stomach was blowing up with gas. The stomach dilates then twists itself in a knot, shutting off the blood supply. And once it's stretched and twisted far enough, the blood from the rear two-thirds of the dog can't get back to the heart. So they go into shock and cardiac failure. About 30 per cent of dogs that get it will die. It used to be 50 per cent. It is a serious emergency that comes out of nowhere.

If you were a vet who didn't do on-call work, you could have an entire career without seeing a single one of these cases, but covering half of South London on the graveyard shift produced plenty. My first one was when an old woman with short hair and big glasses brought in her bull terrier.

'He's dry retching and look at 'is belly. 'E's bloa'ing,' she said.

She was rough around the edges but devoted to her dog and she'd brought him in at the very first sign of trouble. Benny was his name and he was nine years old. She told me he'd got sick a few hours after she'd given him a big feed of dry food.

'Looks like it's a twisted stomach,' I said. 'We can do an X-ray but I think that's just going to confirm what I already suspect. Your dog is very sick. We can save him, but the operation only has a 70 per cent survival rate. So three dogs in ten won't survive it. It's going to cost you about £1200 and we need to make that decision right now. Speed is of the essence.'

This woman, with her short brown curly hair and faded brown coat, clearly did not have a lot of money, but she did not hesitate. 'I love me dog. Let's do i'.'

I sent her home, so it was just Benny, the nurse and I. I got the IV fluids into him to counteract the shock that dogs go into owing to the blood from the back of the body not being able to get back to the heart. I took an X-ray to confirm my diagnosis and then tried to get a stomach tube into his gut to try to get some of the gasses out.

I couldn't work it in there so I proceeded straight to surgery. I made a very large cut along Benny's abdomen, revealing a stomach that was enormously bloated, purple and confused. It was hard to make out exactly which way it had twisted. It felt like it had gone clockwise and statistically I knew that about 75 per cent of them twisted that way. So I grabbed hold of this flaring wine-coloured blob and tried to rotate it gently back counter-clockwise. It was hard to grasp and I wasn't entirely sure I was going in the right direction. Nothing moved at first and I kept doubting myself, fearful that I was making things worse, when all of a sudden the stomach started to move, and then it kept going; the kinetic energy of the twist wound it back into place in the most satisfying of motions. There was an almost instantaneous colour change as the blood started to flow and the whole purple mess subsided to a gentle pink.

I got a tube into the stomach and waited for the gasses and food to come streaming out, but nothing happened. Things were now back in the right spot but the stomach was still hugely bloated. There was no option but to reach for the scalpel again. I opened up the stomach with and found a congealed slurry of grainy rehydrated food that stank of digestive juices.

I cleaned it all out, then set about attaching the stomach to the body by making a small cut in the wall, not all the way through, and a small cut in the body wall, then stitching the two together at the point where the cuts had been made. When the two small cuts healed, the scar tissue would weld them together permanently so the stomach would never twist again. With that done I had to clean up the abdomen and make sure I'd removed all contamination – rushing all the while, because it's been shown that with this operation, the longer you take, the poorer the chance of survival. Animals often die in the aftermath from heart abnormalities that arise out of the huge derangement of their systems that has just taken place. I stitched Benny up as quickly as I could. It was 1 a.m. by now. I let out a huge sigh. What a ride. I woke the dog and he looked great. He went on to be one of the 70 per cent that survive. It's a high-stakes, adrenalin-fuelled procedure that you're doing by yourself in the still of the night. This one was helped by how quickly the owner had brought Benny to us.

I went on to do plenty more. I had a good run there where most of mine were surviving and I allowed myself to think I was becoming a bit of a hot-shot, but unfortunately things have a habit of evening themselves out.

A FIERY REDHEAD

Anthony

Poppy Perkins had her big ginger cat, Willy, out in the waiting room. Willy appeared on edge and probably in pain, but he snuggled in against Poppy as she fondly caressed his chin. 'He's been off his food,' she said, 'and he's been going to the litter box a lot and just squatting there with nothing coming out.'

It wasn't hard to guess what the problem was. When male cats get stressed, they can develop a urinary tract complication that leads to crystals or plugs of mucus forming in their urine. The bladder wall also becomes thickened and inflamed and the damaged cells flake away. A cat's penis is extremely narrow at the tip, so the mucus and flaking cells often block it up. If you don't do something about it, the bladder can fill up till it bursts like a balloon.

'All right, Poppy,' I said, 'I think we're going to have to perform a little operation to unblock this. It's a relatively straightforward procedure. We need to pass a urinary catheter beyond the obstruction and into his bladder to allow him to pass urine freely. We will have to keep him for several nights on a drip with the catheter in place to allow his bladder to settle down and return to normal function.'

Willy was a lovely big gentle fur-ball, but there's something about ginger cats: they seem to have a correlation to fiery redheads. Another thing about cats generally is that when they're in the consult room with their owners, they're gracious and accommodating. They rub on you and purr. It's a pleasure to deal with them. But once you take them through the swinging door to the back of the practice where the operating theatre is, they can turn into balls of pure, unadulterated hatred. Then when you bring them back through those doors to their owner, they revert to normal cats, purring like 1972 Ford Falcons.

Willy was no exception to any of these generalisations. As he went through those doors he arched his back, bristled his fur and frizzed his tail. The slits of his eyes dilated into black circles. When I reached in to pick him up, he showed me the white daggers in his mouth and the talons on his left paw.

He looked so aggressive away from Poppy that there appeared to be no chance of giving him a nice calm intravenous anaesthetic. In such cases, the best practice is to put the cat into a clear plastic box and run anaesthetic through it. Unfortunately, we didn't possess such a box, so we had no choice but to go for a vein.

The nurse, Marie, was really good at it. She reached into the cage and, before Willy knew what had hit him, she had an iron grip on the scruff of his neck and was pulling him out. It's a great skill to be able to do that, then hold the cat's head up and its leg out so it can't readily attack the vet with its back claws. I was able to find a vein and we got Willy knocked out quickly.

Once he was anaesthetised we were able to put a catheter in his penis so he could urinate freely, and we got another one into a vein to provide hydrating fluids and give him painkillers. We kept him in hospital for several days to allow the treatment – antibiotics and anti-inflammatories – a chance to settle things down, before it was time to remove the urinary catheter and send him home. The urinary catheter is only held in place by a single stitch, so it just needs to be nicked and you can pull the catheter out.

As we now know, the underlying cause of this problem is stress, so our treatment regime was somewhat ineffective. Being in a vet clinic with a cone on his head and a catheter in his bladder had done nothing to alleviate the stress that Willy was suffering. Today a lot more drugs are available to relieve anxiety, but ten years ago we were still trying to convince ourselves that the problem was an infection.

Marie and I stood looking at the snarling ball of jagged-toothed ginger wondering what to do. 'Look, I think you're going to have to do the same as last time,' I said. 'There's no way I can get that stitch out without anaesthetising him. He's way too aggressive. You did well last time. Let's see if you can pull it off again today.'

So Marie opened the cage and the moment she put her hand in he went totally berserk. Willy had lost the plot and we had just lost the element of surprise. Marie continued gamely nevertheless, opting for a full-frontal assault. Willy replied with all weapons blazing. Marie got her hands on his neck and scruffed him, but he was a writhing ball of furious elastic and his back feet inflicted a lot of damage on her arms. I came in with a towel to wrap him. Cat wrapping is an expert skill because cats are universally good at unwrapping themselves, generally by shredding the towel – and then you – with their back legs. And that's exactly what Willy did here. He tore that towel to strips. Ditto my arm. And then he started to really go at Marie with his back legs. I went in to help. 'You let go. I'll take it,' I said. I figured we'd get him back in the cage, slam the door shut and rethink our strategy from there.

So I scruffed him, but somehow he turned around and bit me on the hand. Cats have very sharp teeth and they bite very hard. This one got me in the webbing between the thumb and the index finger. But I kept holding on because I knew if I let him go we'd never catch him again. In that moment of intense pain I did find time to wonder how he had managed to bite me. I'd had him by the scruff yet he had been able to spin around and sink his teeth into the very hand that held him. I realised that because he was so big, he had a huge layer of loose skin and that let him turn his head further than other cats. So I gripped it even tighter, but again Willy managed to reach around and bite me. With that electric bolt of pain, my every instinct told me to drop him and run, but I managed to override the impulse and raced to the cage. Then he got me again. Only this time he managed to get a canine tooth into the second joint on my index finger. It felt like someone had put a needle through it. I could no longer override instinct and reflexively shook my hand to flick this 8-kilogram feline away, but its tooth was still in my finger and, as I flicked, the tooth broke all the ligaments in my digit. Any children in the waiting room may have heard some unfamiliar words at a volume that would have broken OH&S decibel limits. Geoff came running.

The cat escaped but we managed to recapture him. We got more helpers and did what we needed to do. The damage, however, had been done to my finger.

Marie put the phone down. 'I've made you an appointment at the doctor. They're waiting for you now.' She was my mother's age and she really looked after me. She knew I probably wouldn't have bothered myself.

Unfortunately the bite had introduced bacteria into the joint and over the next few days it became badly infected. The finger swelled to twice the size of my thumb and then I started to see a red inflammation line move up my arm towards my elbow as the infection spread.

The antibiotics I was on didn't work. It was clear that the germs had come from the cat's mouth, so I wondered if I should use the type of antibiotic that I'd give to a cat with an infected mouth.

I consulted Dad about it. I told him what I wanted to use and he looked it up in a human medical book for me. He said it was cleared for human use but was most commonly used for urinary tract infections. He found the dosage for me and wrote me out a script. About twenty-four hours later the infection was under control.

When my finger had recovered sufficiently for me to fill out a worker's comp form, one of the questions was: 'How soon after the incident did you notify your boss?'

I wrote, 'Three seconds.' Though it may have been less.

Poppy was mortified. She told me that if Willy got another bout of inflammation we'd have to put him to sleep because she wasn't prepared to expose us to the danger any more. There was no way we would have let her do this just for us, but the thought was very much appreciated. To her, Willy was her darling pussy cat who slept in the sun and drank milk. To us, he would always be the monster at the back of the clinic. My finger is aching now just thinking about him.

Willy with the sore willy has gone on to live a long and happy life, I'm told. I've never seen him again. But about four days after the incident, I went out and bought a Perspex box at a $2 shop and made up my own anaesthetic box. Just in case.

DRINKING ON THE JOB

James

One night I was woken by the nurse and told that we had a dog coming in that had swallowed antifreeze. I got up and thought about what I'd need to deal with this emergency. The Jack Russell arrived in the back of a Ford Mondeo station wagon. The owner was a single mum of about forty, with three youngish kids in tow, all in their pyjamas and rubbing sleep from their eyes. She was distressed and a little bedraggled, with her shoulder-length blonde hair all tussled and lank.

'We had him in the back of the wagon where he found the antifreeze,' she said. 'He chewed the top off the plastic bottle and drank it before we knew what was happening.'

'What's the little fellow's name?'

'Keith.'

'Hello, Keith. What have you been eating now?'

For his part, Keith looked fine. The toxic chemicals had not yet produced any symptoms.

'How much did he have?' I asked the owner.

'Most of this bottle,' she said, handing over the bright-green plastic container. 'I couldn't believe the kids didn't tell me. They were like,

"Mum, the dog's drinking the green stuff," and I'm going, "How long's 'e been doing that for?" "A while.'"

Antifreeze is very poisonous to dogs, causing acute kidney failure. It is also sugary and sweet, and therefore tasty and appealing. As the dog had only just drunk it, I could start by trying to get as much out as possible. I did my party trick with the apomorphine under the eyelid to make him vomit, but I knew we'd need to do a lot more. I read on the bottle that ethylene glycol was the active ingredient. I knew that the antidote to ethylene glycol was ethanol, but I didn't have any on hand. I rang the UK's excellent poisons information hotline for animals. The guy on the phone ran me through the rudimentary questions about how much the dog weighed and how much it had eaten.

'Do you have any medical-grade ethanol for injection?' he asked.

'No, we don't.'

'Well, that's what you need. The ethanol outcompetes the ethylene glycol at the binding site so the ethylene glycol gets excreted without damaging the kidney. We need to give it the ethanol intravenously so we can calculate the right dose from the dog's weight.'

'Mate, it's two o'clock in the morning. Where am I going to get some medical grade ethanol?'

'There is another option,' the guy said. 'You can give the dog ethanol orally.'

'Okay?' I didn't see how this solved my problem since I didn't have any ethanol.

'Do you have any really strong alcohol?'

'You mean like booze? For drinking?'

'Yes, booze.'

'Hang on, I'll pop upstairs.'

I ran as quietly as possible up the steep rickety timber steps that we'd dubbed the Stairway to Heaven. Rummaging through the kitchen, I found just the thing and padded back down to the phone. 'Mate, I've got a Smirnoff Black Label vodka that's about 60 per cent alcohol.'

'Okay, great. Let me do some calculations.'

I could hear him tapping away on his calculator, muttering to himself, before he came back on. 'It's good that it's so strong. There are fewer impurities. You're going to have to give the dog ten mils straight away then one mil every fifteen minutes for the next twelve hours.'

'Right, okay.'

'So put it on a drip and give it all the medical care you can. Syringe the vodka in by mouth every fifteen minutes. We've got to keep his ethanol level at that sweet spot.'

Keith's owner was pacing the floor with the dog in her arms when I came back out. I had a quick look at Keith and he still looked ready to go out and destroy some shoes. But I gave it to her straight.

'Keith's looking fine now, but tomorrow he's going to be dead unless we do something. The good news is that I think we can save him. We're going to hook him up to a drip and then we're going to get him drunk.' She looked at me blankly.

I explained it as well as I could then sent her and the kids home. I moved tiny Keith into the biggest cage we had and sat myself down in there with him and the bottle of Smirnoff and a syringe. After about an hour, Keith's face was drooping, but I'm sure he felt like the handsomest, wittiest dog in the world. It was like he was about to start sending texts to ex-girlfriends before streaking down the common. His face went through a range of expressions I wouldn't have thought possible. I was having a jolly good time myself, even though I couldn't join him for a tipple. I had other patients to care for.

I could do the texting, though. I sent a picture of Keith, me and the vodka to the person who'd given it to me as a present and typed PUTTING THE SMIRNOFF TO GOOD USE. My friend didn't mind that I'd given it to a dog. He agreed that saving Keith was more worthwhile than what I was going to use it for.

I love emergency work for its flying-by-the-seat-of-your-pants energy. Often when animals are presented to you they are dying. You've got to get the history, keep the animal alive while examining it, then figure out what's gone wrong and whether it can be saved. It's stressful and sleep depriving, but so rewarding when they walk out of the clinic happy and healthy.

Keith was fairly doughy the next day and really needed a Berocca, a coffee and a bucket of KFC, but we just fed him normally. We had to keep him on a drip for a few days and test his kidney function but he made a full recovery and went home.

The owner bought me a bottle of vodka to replace mine. It was just a cheap no-name brand, but the gesture from someone who was clearly doing it tough was very much appreciated.

THE BERRY SHOWGIRL BALL

Anthony

Barry Alexander wasn't happy. His daughter's pet Brahman cow, Indira, had delivered a stillborn calf then prolapsed. So here he was having to foot my bill on top of there being no prospect of a new calf to offset the cost. And I think Indira had failed to deliver a calf the year before too. Cattle people tend to be hard markers. Cows that don't produce can expect a rigorous dose of truckacillin. But there was no way Barry's daughter was going to let him do that. Indira, with her enormous floppy ears and great folds of dangling skin, was her darling.

Barry was a knockabout type. With not a gram of fat on him, he had arms like Popeye and walked like he was shaping up to punch someone. I hadn't yet got to know Barry and his mood didn't seem exactly conducive to pleasantries. But I still had to do my job and get the uterus back into the cow.

I was on edge about Barry but also about the fact that I was lined up to be master of ceremonies at the Berry Showgirl Ball that night. In a few hours, I would be out of these flyblown overalls and into a tux. I'd never been an MC before and only done a little public speaking, so I was full of nerves. There were going to be a lot of people there. I was mentally running through my speech and thinking about how I'd link up the other speeches and about all the things that could go wrong.

A prolapsed uterus is a difficult job. It's a heavy, slippery mass of purply pink meat covered in black placenta balls that bleed like billy-o if they tear off. Add to this the enormous weight – 30 to 40 kilograms in a big cow – and prolapsed uteri will give a lot of vets the shivers. To get the uterus back into the cow you have to support the weight while carefully finessing the uterus back into the cow and turning it outside in. I had Barry help me by taking the weight of the uterus in his Popeye arms, thereby smearing his well-worn polo shirt with birth juices, while I squeezed the uterus back into the cow. Indira stood calm and patient as we bustled the great bundle of flesh back inside her. It might have taken only fifteen minutes.

The ligaments and muscles that hold a Brahman's uterus in place are a lot looser than in other breeds and hence they tend to prolapse more often, but that also means it's easier to push things back in. I thought there was a strong chance Indira's uterus would fall back out as easily as it had gone in, so I decided we were going to have to staple it in place. I went to the car and brought out an intra-uterine pin. I put my hand into the cow's vagina, covering the spike, then, once inside, I pushed the spike up through the uterus, through the muscles, out through the leathery hide and into daylight. Through all this indignity, Indira remained perfectly still and calm. She had been a poddy calf, hand-raised by Barry's daughter, and was used to humans.

I walked around to her flank and put a cap onto the spike, which was now sticking out her side, securing it in place with a split pin and effectively stapling the uterus to the cow. It can freak people out when they see this great spike coming out the side of their cow. But it does the job.

The operation went well, which was a dangerous sign. Surely Murphy and his law were lurking nearby? It was a hot, humid January day. I was covered in slime, flies and cow poo, but pleased that I'd soon be luxuriating in a cool shower and sprucing up for the night ahead. I cleaned up and gave the cow all the injections she needed while I mentally went through my speech and my jokes one more time. We released Indira's neck from the crush and I bent down to pick up a bucket behind her. As I did so, I saw a flash of light. I thought Barry's watch had reflected the sun towards me, so, as the cow walked away, I looked up at him. But he wasn't looking at his watch; he was looking at me with a horrified expression on his goateed face.

'Did she just try to kick me?' I asked.

'Yep, and she missed you by that much.' His fingers indicated a couple of centimetres.

This cow had stood calmly while I'd perpetrated all those unpleasantries upon her. She had not flinched. She had not complained. But she'd stored it up in her mind. Just when she was free to go, I'd made the mistake of leaning over behind her and she had taken her shot.

But she'd missed. My luck was holding.

Turning up to the Showgirl Ball with a hoof print in my face – or my jaw wired shut or even worse – would not have been a good look. Cow kicks pack a punch. And the look on Barry's face confirmed how lucky I was and how stupid I'd been to put my head in the way of that hoof.

I got home and cleaned up. I pulled the tuxedo out of the dry cleaner's plastic cover and ironed my best white Country Road shirt. The muggy heat hardly let up as the sun went down and all the Berry showgirl contestants gathered in their finery. The ball, as well as being a major date on Berry's social calendar, is a major part of their assessment. The judges watch the contestants throughout the night but particularly while they are being interviewed on stage. One of my main jobs was to introduce them as they came up to be grilled.

The building wasn't air conditioned. I don't know if it was nerves or the bright lights shining into my eyes, but I soon felt like I was the one under the grill. My stiff collar softened with sweat. The circle of moisture under my armpits expanded outwards to annex my entire shirt and my hair went limp as the product that was holding it up surrendered the fight. I don't think I've ever sweated so much. It looked like it was raining in a little circle around me.

But I battled on and was doing okay, introducing the girls as they came up on stage sensibly dressed in their somewhat matronly outfits. I came to a name I recognised, Sidney Roberts, and summoned her forwards. She stood and moved towards the stage in a dazzling, tight-fitting yellow gown with a long train behind her. Aside from a small slip on the stairs when her train got snagged, threatening a major wardrobe derailment, she glided up with a grace I hadn't seen in the others. And on top of being stunningly attractive, she seemed more confident on stage than any of her peers. She mentioned that the exceedingly expensive gown was made out of pineapple husks and had been loaned to her by a friend. I thought she was a certainty to win.

I'd met Sidney once before through some mutual friends but didn't know her at all well. I didn't get a chance to say more than a quick hello to her at the ball. I was up and down all night and she was over at a table with her friends and sponsors. I focused on surviving the ordeal of being an MC. And miraculously, despite the sweat-stained notes and the ever-lurking presence of Murphy, my luck held out.

I went skiing in Japan soon after, so I missed the announcement of the showgirl winner. A day or two after returning home, however, I was walking down the street with one of the new nurses from work, Kahlia, when I saw Sidney sitting outside the Ice Creamery engrossed in her iPad.

As I walked past I waved my hand between her face and the screen to get her attention. She almost went through the roof with fright. I felt like a total clod. 'Oh God, I'm sorry,' I said. But because I was walking with Kahlia, I couldn't really stop to talk.

'We should catch up for dinner,' I called out over my shoulder. 'You can tell me how the showgirl competition went.'

'That'd be lovely,' she said.

I made the international sign language symbol for the telephone with my thumb and little finger and that was it. It was a date. Only it wasn't a date. There was none of the usual nervousness on my part that I'd normally feel asking a girl out for the first time because I really didn't see it as a date. As far as I knew she had a boyfriend. It was not a romantic thing. It was just a catch-up. Really.

Nevertheless, I was cautious when I rang her to tee it up. 'Maybe it's best we don't have dinner in town,' I said. 'It'd get misconstrued if people see us together. Small town and all that. How about we get some takeaway Thai and take it down to the beach?'

'That sounds lovely,' she said again.

We did that. I brought along some bowls, forks, a bottle of white wine and some plastic soft-drink cups. Just as we started to tuck into the spring rolls, out of the surf came Brad Tregonning, walking straight past us with his long board and longer smile. You might describe Brad's mum, Shirley, as 'well connected'. I knew that if Brad told her what he'd seen, she'd have her megaphone handy and soon the whole town would be seeing our little picnic as something totally different from what it was. Despite my concerns, though, we had a very pleasant evening and as darkness fell we packed up and I drove Sidney home. On the way, I asked, by the by, 'How's your boyfriend going?'

'I don't have a boyfriend,' she replied casually. 'We broke up months ago.' The words hit me like a sledgehammer. No longer was there any road noise, I couldn't hear the radio and my vision seemed to be coning down onto the road. I was in my own little world, nothing was getting in. I was focused on processing the immensity of that statement. I somehow managed to indicate right and turned the ute onto Beach Road, then the reality of the situation sank in: *Oh my God! This is a date!*

I had honestly thought it was an innocent catch-up. But what had Sidney been thinking? She must have thought it was a date. And yet she had accepted. I had actually asked a stunningly beautiful girl out on a date without experiencing any of the nerves usually associated with such a task.

I took Sidney back to her parents' farm and we ended up chatting for hours. When I got home I couldn't get her or the whole misconception thing out of my head. It churned away between my belly and my brain. I couldn't sleep for hours. It rumbled along all day Saturday as I worked through what was going on and what everybody was going to think was going on. But when I woke up on Sunday morning there was a certain clarity. *If that wasn't a date yet everybody thinks it was, I might as well try to have one.* I picked up the phone with a distinct lack of adrenalin. Even though I might fret over a problem for a long time, once I've decided that a course of action is the correct way to go, I tend to follow it through without further ado. Be it surgery or a touch-footy grand final, I tend to dive in and get on with it.

So I asked Sidney out to dinner again. And again she said yes. There was just the matter of where to have it.

'I know it's not kosher to have someone over to your house on a second date,' I continued, 'but it's probably better to go to your place or mine to avoid any unhelpful scrutiny.'

'Yes, I know what you mean.'

'How about I cook tea for you?' I offered.

'That would be lovely,' she said a third time.

I made zucchini conchiglie – a dish of little sea-shell pastas with a lot of oil, parmesan and zucchini. I broke open a flash bottle of red and a pack of candles that I had in reserve in case the power went off.

I knew they weren't the little romantic tea-light ones, but I figured a candle was a candle.

Anyway, it all went well. That's where the romance started. And I realised that if that kick back at Barry Alexander's place had connected it might have changed my destiny. She might not have liked a punch-drunk bloke with a hoof print in his face.

My luck had continued to hold.

STITCHING THINGS BACK TOGETHER

James

After two and a half years in London having a great time, Ronnie and I both had a feeling that it was time to go home, grow up and get a haircut and a real job. Before we did that though, we bought a campervan, Trevor the Transit Van, and headed off for a big European adventure. We got as far east as the Czech Republic and Croatia and then did a bit of ferry hopping along the Mediterranean.

Secreted inside some camera equipment in the van's safe was a diamond ring. When we got to Sardinia we hired a boat for a day. I think Ronnie knew something was afoot when I didn't baulk at the €200 rental fee. We motored through crystal-clear blue waters to a deserted cove and swam ashore to a sandy white beach. I made her sit atop a beautiful rock before pulling the ring from my boardies and popping the question.

She said yes.

And so it was that we returned to Australia engaged. I'd been away for three and a half years and Ronnie just a little less. We'd had the adventure and now it was time to get on with the next stage of life. For me, that meant owning my own business. It was just a matter of saving money and awaiting the right opportunity. In the meantime

I began a master's degree in small-animal practice and got a job at the Ku-Ring-Gai Veterinary Hospital. It was very high-end, with nine vets, visiting specialists and human-grade operating facilities. It had a CT machine in the basement. The caseload was enormous, and they worked us hard.

When I was on the 7 a.m. shift, I'd arrive in the morning and there'd be up to forty animals that needed to be examined before 8 a.m. Two nurses would walk the animals out to me and I'd look at them and tweak their treatment plans. It was more like a human hospital in that doctors dispensed instructions and nurses carried them out. Then the day would really crank up with new patients rolling in. You had the facilities to manage cases much more intensively and thoroughly. It was tremendously busy and the hours were long, but it was great exposure to that type of care.

Among the many cases I handled at Ku-Ring-Gai, one stood out. A lovely German shepherd cross called Foster was brought in by a mother and her young-adult son. They explained that Foster had been vomiting a couple of days earlier and they'd taken him to an emergency vet who'd wanted to run some tests but they hadn't thought it necessary. So they'd gone home and Foster had initially improved. But now he was vomiting again.

I had a look at Foster and he seemed like a bright-eyed, friendly dog. A skin pinch revealed he was a little dehydrated. I pressed into his abdomen and he flinched, indicating pain, but he instantly reverted to being a tongue-out happy feller when I took the pressure off. He wasn't going to let a bit of pain ruin his chance to enjoy all this attention.

He was eight years old, so I thought a tumour was a possibility. I rearranged my schedule and told the owners to come back in a couple of hours. I gave Foster some pain relief, then shaved his abdomen from his sternum up to his spinal muscles and back down his belly. I rubbed off the last of his hair and prepped the skin with metho to improve the contact with the ultrasound machine before applying the gel and gently running the probe over his belly.

I couldn't find any lumps, but what I did see was a lot of fluid and a 'plicated' intestine. That means the sausage-like intestine has folded up on itself; it typically looks like a collapsed fan. I had a strong suspicion of what was wrong.

When the owners returned, I asked, 'Is he the sort of dog that'll eat anything in sight?'

'No, not that we're aware of. He's usually pretty good like that.'

'Has he been playing with string or something similar?'

'No. Don't think so.'

'Well, from what I'm seeing in the ultrasound, it's looking like he might have swallowed a piece of string.' I saw their faces brighten and nod with hope. Surely something so simple could easily be fixed?

But I had to explain that Foster was in trouble. 'It's what we vets call a linear foreign body, and I'm afraid I've got to tell you that linear foreign bodies are particularly awful. When a length of string lodges in the stomach and some of it goes down the intestine, that's when you get into real strife. I think that's what we've got here.' They nodded in silence, but I knew they didn't quite get how it could be so dangerous.

'The intestine is a long tube designed to steadily move things along its length,' I continued. 'When the string lodges in the stomach, the intestine tries to push it along but it can't. So the intestine bunches up like when you're trying to thread a cord into your swimming cossies. Then, because it can't move the string along, it remains in that folded position with the string running straight through it. Eventually the string saws through the intestine and perforates it.'

'So what are our options?' the mother asked.

'Basically, we need to open this dog up to assess what's going on. If it is a linear foreign body stuck in there, it needs prompt attention because left untreated it will kill him.'

'And what guarantee is there that the operation will work?'

'There's no guarantee that it will save him. Foster is in a lot of trouble, but, if he does survive, he will make a full recovery. He's only eight, so he's got a lot of good years ahead of him.'

We discussed costs and the mother and son talked briefly before the mother came back to me. 'I've got to call my ex-husband. It's his dog too and I think we all need to be in on this.'

The son got on the phone to his sister and they had a big four-way conference before coming back to me. 'We want you to do whatever you need to do to save Foster.'

It was mid-afternoon and luckily it was a day when my colleague Jill was working. Jill had done a surgery residency and her role in the clinic was to perform very difficult operations, just like this one. She looked at the ultrasound with me.

'He's been vomiting for a few days?' she asked.

I nodded.

'I don't like the look of this at all. I can't believe this dog isn't sicker.'

We opened Foster up. The first thing we saw was raging peritonitis – infection of the abdomen. We pushed on, down to the suspected root of the problem, where the stomach meets the intestine. I cut into the stomach, revealing a mat of brown string-like material, stained heavily with bile, plugging the stomach's exit hole. I snipped the mat away and instantly we saw the tension come off the concertinaed intestine. But as the bends softened out, they revealed a line of dashes along the intestine wall where the string had cut through. And we knew there'd be a corresponding line of dashes on the underside that we couldn't see.

So we set about the laborious task of cutting out the bits of intestine that were worst affected, some of which were rotting away. We couldn't take out all of the diseased sections, otherwise the dog would have been left with almost no small intestine, but we nevertheless took out an enormous amount. The surgery lasted hours, and we did all that we could. Suturing, suturing, suturing, making sure that nothing was leaking. It was a marathon, and there were several moments when Jill and I thought we couldn't go on, but we kept at it and got everything back together. By the time we finished, the gut was a lot shorter, and then we stitched the rest of poor old Foster back together. I woke him up and for all the world he was a new dog. Bright and alert and even more friendly than before. I allowed myself to hope that we'd done enough.

At first, Foster recovered well. He began to eat a little and keep it down. But a few days later a nurse walked him in to me on the 7 a.m. round. His tail wagged and his head lifted when he saw me, but that couldn't hide a general flatness in his demeanour. 'He hasn't eaten in twenty-four hours and his temperature is up,' the nurse said.

It was likely that at least one of the surgery sites was breaking down, releasing infection and digestive material into the cavity of the abdomen. So I ultrasounded him again on his still-shaven belly and the infection was plain to see. This was a massive problem, and one that could only be fixed with more surgery.

I rang the owners and more four-way conferencing ensued. I explained that we had to do another operation to remove the failed section of gut. When Jill and I opened the abdomen we were again up against a massive amount of peritonitis and infection, but now we could see that there was only one area that was causing the problem. We cut it out and stitched the ever-decreasing intestine back together. The operation was a success and the intestine held.

Foster again showed an immediate improvement, but he was still sick. He remained flat and we could tell the infection was still in there. By this stage it was a massive inflammatory and infectious process in his abdomen. We had fixed the problem, but the dog was being consumed by the peritonitis.

Foster stayed in the hospital. While we fought to save this beautiful, brave dog, he never gave a hint that he was unhappy. During the weeks he was with us, his complete obliviousness to his own misfortune won over all those who came into his orbit. For all his problems he seemed to possess a saintly glow. We did plasma transfusions and blood transfusions. We gave him antibiotics then more antibiotics, even as the infection continued to consume him. Drains protruded from his belly to draw the infected fluid away. And all the while his tail wagged and his eyes sparkled.

As our treatment regime ballooned, so too did the family's bill. We informed them of the costs all the way. They kept liaising with each other and they kept telling us to keep going. They poured their hearts into this dog. They were always in there visiting him, usually separately because the parents were divorced and the kids were off leading their own lives, but they'd often bump into each other by his side. The dog was their touchstone.

The bill ticked up over $8000 and, after another of their family conferences, the father rang in to tell me they just couldn't keep going. They couldn't afford any more.

I knew how they felt. I'd had my own financial limitations when I'd needed to treat Toby the Wonder Dog, and I'd really fallen for Foster too. I explained the situation to my bosses, who had also been won over by this happy dog who seemed so impervious to pain and misery. So they gave me the go-ahead to keep fighting free of charge.

Foster continued to wag his tail when he saw me and he continued to perk up and get that spark in his eye, but he never quite recovered. One morning I came in on my 7 a.m. rounds and saw that Foster's belly seemed more swollen than before. The fluids produced by the infection were getting out of hand. Later in the morning, when I found a minute, I ultrasounded the wound and saw the inflammation was even worse.

The father had rung in the morning and said that he was coming in for a visit, so I waited for his arrival to deliver the bad news. I had Foster up on a table, where his belly bulged like a pregnant sow.

'I think we're at a stage where we're not going to win here. We need to think about putting Foster to sleep.'

'Yes, I think the same, but I'd better call my children and my ex-wife.'

So I left him to it and went back to type up my notes. Then I saw the father waving me over. I walked up to the table, and Foster was dead. The father told me that he had slipped away while the family were all agreeing to end his pain. 'I was patting him when he looked up, wagged his tail and went to sleep.' Dogs usually die gasping for air or struggling to hold onto that last glimmer of life. They don't die connected and peaceful, as humans often do. Foster remains the only dog I've ever heard of that went like that.

The family all came in and they cried. It was the culmination of a huge amount of effort and stress.

'Oh, James, thank you so much for all your efforts,' the mother said, barely containing her tears.

'I only wish there was something more we could have done,' I said, grateful to receive their thanks but acutely aware of that hollow feeling you get when you're standing over the body of a dead pet. Particularly one as special as Foster. Pets are always special to their owners, but it doesn't always cut through to the vet. Foster, however, had cut through. And here he was in death bringing this family, who had gone their separate ways, back together.

They lingered with him for a long time, not saying much. I went off and busied myself nearby. I overheard the man talking to his ex-wife and all the kids.

'How 'bout we get something to eat?' he said.

'Yes, I'd like that,' said the ex-wife, and the children chorused in agreement.

TOAST IN THE PAST AND TOAST
TO THE FUTURE

Anthony

At uni, our group of friends had spent every day moving from class to class with each other. Then in fourth year we'd all lived together at Camden as well as going to all the same classes. We played sport, partied, mucked up and ate Toasted Bread Sandwiches together. It got to the point where we didn't even wash alone. You'd hear someone coming past your room. 'I'm going for a shower, you coming?'

'Yeah.'

You'd knock on the next door. 'You been for a shower yet?'

'Nah, you got the drinks?' We'd all be in the cubicles chatting away through the steam.

Suddenly it was all over and everybody went their separate ways. I found it quite tough. In those early years, we'd reconvene in Sydney every month or two, driving from all over the place. It was still a tight group. Over time, however, the catch-ups became less frequent. We clung to one tradition, though – spending a day or two each summer at a cricket Test.

We tried to go to a different city every year. In 2010, Australia was playing England and we'd all gathered in Brisbane for the first Test.

Australia had bundled England out on the first day for 280 but, like us vets, was looking a little patchy in reply on the second day. I was sitting next to James in the sun, a plastic cup of light beer in hand, when I asked him, 'What are your plans down the track? What do you think you're gunna do?'

'We're staying in Australia but, yeah, I don't know. I don't really want to stay in Sydney. Ultimately I want my own practice.'

'You should think about coming to Berry. Geoff's going to be retiring soon. It's a great work–life balance and a great mixture of work, if you want to go back into mixed practice, that is.'

'Mate, if it was up to me I'd be there tomorrow. But it's Ronnie's call too. She's grown up in the city and never lived in the country. I'm not sure how she'd handle it.'

Towards the end of that summer, I was hosting a party at Dad's place in the city, when James pulled me aside. 'Mate, can I have a word with you outside on the balcony?' The party was really happening, there were people everywhere. He had a bottle of champagne in his hand. Ronnie followed us out. 'We've talked about it and decided we would like to come to Berry if we can make it work,' James said, wrestling with the champagne cork.

'Oh, mate, that's fantastic,' I said, as the cork popped and flew into the darkness.

'So let's make this happen,' he said, pouring. 'Let's make it work. Here's to our lives together.'

The three of us toasted the future.

PRACTICE MAKES PERFECT

James

Every year the University of Sydney puts on a free conference for all the vet clinics that take students for prac work. In 2006, when I was working at Barraba, I got to go along for some continuing education.

A lot of the vets there were quite a bit older than me, so I gravitated towards Peter Alexander, a vet from Bega who'd taken me in for prac work. I was chatting with him when he introduced me to his mate from Berry, Geoff Manning. I knew Geoff was Anthony's boss so we had a good old chat.

As with any such educational gathering, we went out for a few beers, and then a few more. If there was one thing that stood out about Geoff it was how good he was at convincing the drug company sales reps that it was in their interest to buy us beers, dinner and just about anything. So I ended up at the Nag's Head in Glebe with Geoff, the drug reps, Peter Alexander and Kym Hagon, the vet who later replaced me at Manilla. The drug rep was getting tired and Geoff foresaw a financial crisis. But he managed to persuade the rep to foot the bill for the rest of the night even if he didn't stay. Of course, we didn't abuse the privilege and we felt fine for the next day of the conference. Up and at 'em.

The next night, Geoff's wife, Pauline, and Pete's wife, Mandy, came to the conference's formal dinner and we sat there in our crisp suits and ties like it was a bird surgery exam. Geoff was full of ideas, and one was that it would be a great idea if I came to Berry and went into partnership with Anthony. He was suturing all those loose ends of his life. I let his flippant plans for my future flutter away with the breeze. Geoff was still in his fifties, and I didn't even know his daughter. It was all very far-fetched.

Fast-forward four years, though, and the perspective had changed.

As blokes, you don't tend to pick up the phone to have a chat. Our annual Test match reunion, on the other hand, was great for checking in with what everyone was doing and talking about how good you used to be. Hussey and Haddin were destroying the Poms on their way to a 300-run partnership when Anthony asked me what my plans were.

I told him we were back in the country for good and that I was looking for something to buy into. Then I asked him what was happening at Berry now that Geoff was nearing retirement age. 'What are you planning to do?'

'I was intending to buy it from Geoff,' he said, 'but I'm not sure I want to run the whole thing by myself. It's a matter of finding the right person.'

'What about me?' I said, taking a sip from my plastic cup of beer. 'What do you reckon?'

I'd like to think that a Mexican wave went around at this exact moment or that I at least got to punch a beach ball away from approaching security guards as Anthony answered.

'Maaaaaate, that'd be great. Maybe I should put you in contact with Geoff for a chat.'

It was a long process. Ronnie and I had to discuss whether it was something we wanted to do. For me, it was about going back to mixed practice, which had always been my preference. But we were getting married and had bought an apartment and renovated. To leave it all and move to the country was a huge shift, especially for Ronnie. She'd grown up in the city and the work she could do there was different from what she could find in Berry. On the other hand, we'd set a date for our wedding and were planning to get cracking on the business of having a baby very soon. Life was about to change for us regardless. So we just had to choose how much.

My only experience of that part of the NSW South Coast was doing prac work at Anthony's dad's farm. I knew Berry was a pretty little town, a country retreat for city folk, and that was about it.

So Ronnie and I spent a couple of weekends staying at Anthony's place to test drive the town. On one of them, we spent a spectacular couple of days enjoying the last weekend of my twenties, visiting the wineries and restaurants that Berry had to offer. While there, we weighed up our options. We thought about buying into a Sydney practice or even starting our own. But Berry just seemed like the best way to go – how could we say no? It was truly a beautiful spot. Once we'd decided it was our preferred option, we told Anthony during a party at his dad's place, and then we spoke to Geoff.

I had to come to terms with Geoff and figure out when he wanted to go, and we had to organise a loan and the contracts. It was a long process, during which Ronnie and I married and Ronnie fell pregnant.

In June 2012, some twenty months after the cricket game, we made the move. We rented a little house ten minutes away from Berry, at Gerroa, a village that straddles a headland jutting into the Pacific Ocean. Our house was a tiny brick place right on the promontory, designed as if its million-dollar view didn't exist – you had to stand on the toilet to look down Seven Mile Beach, with all its misty moods and magic sunsets. Nevertheless, the location and the view reinforced the idea that there was so much magic out there if you could just extricate yourself from the rat race to find it.

The very first day I worked at Berry, I got home at about 6 p.m. and was alone because Ronnie was still working in Sydney and staying at our flat in Manly. It was already dark and I opened the door for Bailey to go into the backyard. She immediately waddled onto the grass and started barking.

'What's up, Bailey?'

She was agitated, trying to tell me something was awry. She was fixated on the ocean and kept barking as she edged closer to it in the manner of fraidy-cat dogs.

'What are you doing, Bailey? What are you barking at?'

I looked out to the ocean and there, probably thirty metres from where the backyard ended, I saw a dark shape wallowing in the moonlight. Then it breathed a snorting breath. It was a whale, and Bailey wasn't happy about it.

'It's okay, Bailey. It's okay.' She wagged her tail and came over for a pat as I realised that a mother and calf were out there kicking around, tails breaching. *Wow! What a spot.*

The next night I went to Geoff and Pauline's place for dinner. A neighbour was there too. 'Did you see the whale last night?' they said.

'Yeah, I did. Amazing.'

'Unbelievable how close it was. Honestly, we've lived here forty years and I've never seen one that close before.'

'I've been here one day and I expect whales at my back door every night for the duration. Anything less and I'm moving.'

There were no more whales, but to have been able to plonk myself on the back lawn and enjoy that show reinforced the feeling that there was a certain magic to the area. It has continued to deliver metaphorical whales ever since.

UP TO OUR ARMPITS AGAIN

Anthony

We knew that going into business might spoil a good friendship. But we figured that wasn't a good enough reason not to do it. Knowing someone as well as we knew each other gave us a better understanding of how the other worked. We were the same age, had the same teaching and similar values. It had to be a good start.

All my life I'd worked with guys who were much older than me. The Geoffs had children who were my age, so those relationships had been more like a father–son thing. We'd never gone for a drink on a Friday afternoon. So it was quite refreshing, the first Friday of being in business together, when James asked, 'You want to go for a beer?'

It was a nice way to end the week. It was exciting to work with someone with the same ambitions and same desire to build the practice; somebody who was at the same stage of life, trying to make ends meet while putting things in place for down the track.

We thought we'd get on okay, but we didn't realise how synergistic the working relationship would be. We've both got our own strengths, yet we share ideals and a work ethic. It was still just the two of us working the whole practice, though, so we could hardly say that we'd got the work–life balance right.

First up, we renovated the Berry clinic. We'd be in at 5 a.m. doing paperwork or working on the renovations. We'd do the full day's rounds and then through the evening we'd tackle all the things we hadn't been able to get to during the day – ultrasounding, X-raying, fixing broken legs. The nurses couldn't hang around late, so we'd do a lot of stuff together. Sidney and Ronnie might come in to meet us for dinner. We'd walk down the street and eat, then the two of us would go back to work while the girls went home.

As soon as the renovation was finished, we began work on opening a new clinic in Shoalhaven Heads. It started out as a large bare room. We had the walls put in, the lights and power and a special floor. We painted it ourselves. It was the middle of winter, freezing cold. We'd be in there at 5 a.m. with a single bare light on an extension cord to light the whole place. The fog of our breath impeded the view of our work. If stress was ever going to crack the partnership, this was when it was most likely to happen.

'When we need to redo the next clinic,' I said, almost up to my armpits in a paint tin, 'we're paying painters. This is the last bloody vet clinic I'm painting.'

'Done,' James said. 'It's a deal.'

ACKNOWLEDGEMENTS

We hope that you have as much fun reading this book as we had writing it. Mark Whittaker is a great friend and client and we thank him for helping us transpose our stories onto paper – we both looked forward to our afternoon sessions telling our stories to Mark – and not once did he make us feel that this was just a job for him. Thanks for all your work! Let it be said that Mark is much better at faking interest than our wives!

This book would never have happened without the vision and commitment of Brigitta Doyle, Kate Mayes and Mary Rennie from ABC/HarperCollins. Their passion for this project from the very beginning is what got the book off the ground and it has been an absolute pleasure working with them all.

Of course, our lives changed dramatically when the one and only, the whirlwind, the phenomenon that is Rodney Richmond walked through the Berry Vet Clinic doors some three years ago now and initiated what would one day become *Village Vets*. What started as an idea soon became a pilot and, in the hands of Screentime and Foxtel, a television series. Rod's mateship and dedication have been unwavering.

Thank you also to Simone Landes for helping guide us through the wild media world and for putting up with our rowdy conversation and unfunny jokes on a weekly basis – we can appreciate why you don't like conference calls.

Thank you to everyone that has helped us in our careers, and especially the vets who took the gamble to employ us as the new green graduates we were. Ben Gardiner, Geoff Manning and Geoff Scarlett, you taught, supported and mentored us in our formative first few years in the profession and continue to do so today.

The vets and nurses that we have worked with, worked for and met through our profession have all helped shape us as vets and people, and we are immensely proud to be part of the veterinary profession.

Thanks to our wonderful clients, friends and their animals in Berry and beyond. We may live in the best part of the most privileged country in the world, yet dealing with lovely people every day makes our work so much more fun. Your commitment to your pets and livestock never ceases to amaze us and we thank you for involving and trusting us with your animals' care.

The Berry Vet Clinic staff and their families deserve a particularly big thank you. Our workplace is a lot like a family and your hard work is much appreciated. You keep the ship afloat when we are gallivanting around the countryside and further afield. We cannot thank you enough for your professionalism and friendship, and it makes coming to work every day a pleasure.

Thank you to our wives, Sidney Bennett and Veronica Carroll. You both knew you were marrying vets but we bet you didn't expect this. We appreciate your unwavering support and constructive criticism, but mainly your unwavering support. We know we work long hours and we both wish we were home a lot more often with our families. We probably occasionally come home a bit grumpy but we hope you know that we are doing it all for you – we love you both very much.

Thank you to our parents for raising us in such a caring and nurturing manner and endlessly encouraging us to keep working hard.

Without the support of our parents and siblings we could never have survived our high school and university days, and undoubtedly our careers would be significantly different.

While clearly not an instructional manual on how to be a vet, we hope that this gives people an insight into what it's like to be in a mixed-practice, and that vets and aspiring vets can relate to the stories and the fun and variety of challenges we are privileged to experience every day!

—